Disclaimer (Exclusive clause)

The author and all employees disclaim any incorrect interpretation, wrong answers to questions or text, harm, including emotional, psychological, and physical or any form of the liability to the reader/listener or being Given information by third parties.

Furthermore, this disclaimer protects all contributory people, directors, employees, 3rd parties, authors and will not be liable for any injury caused.

Summary Content

Contents

Dedication

I dedicate this book to myself, to appreciate the hard work that has enabled me to achieve so much, thanks to the blessings of God.

Acknowledgement.

As with all the 160 books I have written and published, I acknowledge the guidance, wisdom, and knowledge that Almighty God provided me through the Guardians in drafting this book. It would have been impossible to finish authoring these books because when I started writing,

I never knew how or when I would conclude my research or where to direct it, but once I began, I received more guidance from Almighty God. With him, this book was written. He produced and gave me the resources; therefore, the real author of this publication is God.

Forgive and love everyone, then trust, believe, and have faith in God. This FORMULA IS THE KEY TO HEAVEN.

Preface

This book covers a wide range of nursing dissertation topics, including

Variety of Veterinary Illnesses, Drug Side Effects (Vancomycin), Research Ethics Practices, Cybersecurity Risks in Healthcare, Addison's Disease, Trauma and Emergency Nursing. The last chapter has more questions and Answers

General nursing is a foundational aspect of healthcare that plays a critical role in patient care, education, and health promotion across various settings. General nurses are essential in ensuring that patients receive comprehensive and compassionate care throughout their healthcare journey.

Nursing is a safety-critical profession founded on four pillars: clinical practice, education, research, and leadership.

General nursing encompasses the practice of nursing that does not specialise in a specific area of healthcare. General nurses, often referred to as registered nurses (RNs) or licensed practical nurses (LPNs), provide essential care to patients in various settings, including hospitals, clinics, nursing homes, and community health centres. Their role is crucial in promoting health, preventing illness, and managing patient care.

General nurses have a wide range of responsibilities, which include:

Patient Assessment: Evaluating patients' health status by taking vital signs, observing symptoms, and identifying changes in their condition.

Medication Administration: Administering prescribed medications and ensuring proper dosages and timing.

Basic Care: Providing essential care such as dressing wounds, assisting with daily activities, and monitoring patient progress.

Patient Education: Educating patients and their families about health conditions, treatment plans, and self-care strategies. Care Coordination: Collaborating with other healthcare professionals to ensure comprehensive patient care. Record Keeping: Maintaining accurate patient records, including health status and treatment plans.

About the Author

My life experience, from being an abandoned child who ate from bins and gutters in Ghana to becoming one of the most successful businessmen in Europe. My first profession is a qualified psychiatric nurse.

I have visited most European countries and wish to share my experiences with my readers. I have also written over 160 books and hold numerous qualifications, which are listed at the end of this book.

I hold approximately six degrees, including four postgraduate qualifications, ten diplomas and 15 certificates.

All are listed in this book.

DETAIL CONTENT

CONTENT

CONTENT

Chapter 2

An investigation into drug side effects (Vancomycin)

Content

Chapter 3

An Overview of Research Ethics Practices

Content

Chapter 4

Importance of Carrying Around Devices to Reduce Cybersecurity Risks in Healthcare.

Content

1. Discuss the advantages and risks of using portable devices in healthcare.
2. Explain how the five steps of the cybersecurity framework (from the textbook) apply to using portable devices and help manage risk.
3. Overall, do you agree or disagree with using portable devices in healthcare? Why or why not?

References

Chapter 7

Addison Disease

Content

Chapter 8

Trauma and Emergency Nursing questions

Content

1. Severe facial injuries, for example, those resulting from going through a windshield, increase the risk for all of the following. For which complication would you assess first?

2. Which drug treatment helps to decrease ICP by expanding plasma and the osmotic effect of moving fluid?

How It Works:

Signs and symptoms

Observing

3. Application of RICE (rest, ice, compression, and elevation) is indicated for initial management of which type of injury?

Breakdown of RICE for Injury Management

Examples of Injuries Where RICE is Applied

Limitations of RICE

4. You are performing abdominal thrusts on a 9-year-old child when he suddenly becomes unresponsive. After you shout for help from nearby, what is the most appropriate action to take?

1. Call for Emergency Help
2. Lay the Child on a Flat Surface
3. Check for Breathing and Pulse
4. Initiate Chest Compressions
5. Give Rescue Breaths

6. Check for Foreign Objects in the Mouth

Chapter 9

Trauma

Content

Priority Decision:

During the primary survey, the nurse identified asymmetric chest wall movement in the patient. What intervention should the nurse first perform?

Immediate First Intervention:

Administer Supplemental Oxygen

Additional Steps Based on Findings

Call for Emergency Assistance

Prepare for Intubation or Mechanical Ventilation (If Necessary)

Perform Needle Decompression for Suspected Tension Pneumothorax

Assist with Chest Tube Insertion

Immobilise Flail Chest (If Applicable)

Continuous Monitoring

Rationale

Why must the nurse obtain details of the incident during the secondary survey of a trauma patient in the Emergency Department?

a) Guiding Focused Assessment and Treatment

Chapter 10

Veterans Access to Care Department of Veterans Affairs Health Care.

Content

Chapter 11

Nursing Q & A

Content

When a pulse is present, how often should rescue breaths be given in infants and children? One breath every 2 to 3 seconds.

Priority Decision: Triage the following patient situations that may be present in an emergency department (ED) as 1, 2, 3, 4, or 5 on the Emergency Severity Index.

Patient Situation 1: 35-year-old male presenting with chest pain and diaphoresis

- Triage Level: ESI 2

Patient Situation 2: 28-year-old woman with a severe asthma exacerbation, speaking in one-word sentences and using accessory muscles to breathe

- Triage Level: ESI 1

Patient Situation 3: 50-year-old man with acute abdominal pain radiating to the back, vomiting, and diaphoresis

- Triage Level: ESI 2

Patient Situation 4: 67-year-old woman with a cough, fever, and body aches for two days

- Triage Level: ESI 4

Patient Situation 5: 25-year-old man with a laceration to the hand after cutting himself with a kitchen knife, controlled bleeding

- Triage Level: ESI 5

When a nurse performs a primary survey in the ED, what is she assessing?

A - Airway with Cervical Spine Protection

B - Breathing

C - Circulation with Haemorrhage Control

Disability (Neurological Status)

E - Exposure/Environmental Control

Additional Considerations in the Primary Survey

Chapter 12

An Overview of Research Ethics Practices

Content

Chapter 1

An Extensive Analysis Investigating the Wide Variety of Veterinary Illnesses

CONTENT

An Extensive Analysis Investigating the Wide Variety of Veterinary Illnesses.

Veterinary medicine leads the way in providing advanced treatment for animals by addressing a broad spectrum of disorders that affect various animal species. Veterinarians treat a wide range of conditions that require careful diagnosis and treatment, including congenital, infectious, metabolic, and neoplastic disorders (Stoewen et al., 2019). This research paper provides the reader with an overview of ten distinct illnesses that affect various animal species, including dogs, cats, horses, pigs, and exotic animals. Every disease presents additional obstacles to overcome, necessitating a multifaceted strategy that encompasses prevention, treatment, diagnosis, and control. We aim to shed light on the agents responsible for species vulnerability, clinical presentation, modes of diagnosis, therapeutic approaches, prophylactic measures, vaccination schedules, zoonotic potential, and containment strategies for contagious diseases in veterinary settings.

Canine Disease

Contagious/Infectious Rabies

The rabies virus primarily affects dogs, especially indoor pets, and is the leading cause of rabies worldwide. After it reaches the central nervous system, people may experience altered behaviour, paralysis, or even death. Humans are among the mammals that can get rabies. The clinical signs include paralysis, increased salivation, aggression, and difficulty swallowing (World Health Organisation, 2019). Diagnostic tests, such as RT-PCR and the Direct Fluorescent Antibody test, are used. The prognosis for rabies is dire; once clinical symptoms manifest, there is sadly no treatment, and euthanasia is advised. Prevention involves vaccinations, wildlife control, and raising awareness to prevent the spread of diseases. Typically, vaccination techniques entail injecting dead viral vaccines intramuscularly. Improper administration or storage might lead to problems. Considering its zoonotic potential, workplace safety precautions are essential (Rupprecht et al.,

2017). Contagious illness transmission is halted by isolation, vaccination, and quarantine.

Borreliosis or Lyme Disease.

The illness primarily affects dogs and is primarily caused by the bacterium Borrelia burgdorferi, which is often carried by ticks. Fever, loss of appetite, lameness, and swollen joints are among the symptoms. Renal illness and persistent joint inflammation are possible outcomes. People are among the other mammals that might be affected. Clinical signs include fever, joint discomfort, enlarged lymph nodes, and lethargy (O'Brien et al., 2021). Several diagnostic assays that aid in diagnosis include Western blot, ELISA, and PCR. When treated with antibiotics like doxycycline, the prognosis is favourable if the illness is discovered early. Prevention includes managing tick populations, getting vaccinated against tick-borne diseases, and avoiding areas infested with ticks. Vaccination for dogs is available; however, complications may occur. Given its zoonotic potential, preventive measures include avoiding ticks and promptly removing them. Contagious spread is mitigated through the use of tick control products and regular inspections.

Feline Diseases

Degenerative/Idiopathic: Feline Lower Urinary Tract Disease (FLUTD).

Several variables, including stress, diet, and environment, can exacerbate feline lower urinary tract disease (FLUTD), a complex condition affecting cats. Urinary difficulties (dysuria), blood in the urine (hematuria), frequent urination, and vocalisations are all caused by inflammation in the bladder and urethra (Astuty et al., 2020). Nephrolysis, imaging, and occasionally urine culture are used in the diagnosis process. The primary objectives of treatment are stress reduction, nutrition changes, and pain alleviation. The prognosis depends on the severity and recurrence of the condition. While not contagious, multicat families can prevent epidemics by minimising stress and maintaining cleanliness (Nivy et al., 2019). Vaccination against other feline diseases is advised even if there is no specific vaccine for this illness.

Toxic: Lead Toxicity

Cats who eat things polluted with lead can get lead poisoning, which is a dangerous ailment.

Seizures, ataxia, weakness, vomiting, and diarrhoea are typical symptoms. X-rays, urine analysis, and blood lead level testing are used to make the diagnosis. Lead removal from the body is achieved by chelation therapy (Altınok-Yipel et al., 2022). The severity of exposure and the extent of organ damage determine prognosis. Remove lead sources, dispose of trash properly, and inform pet owners about the risks of lead poisoning to prevent exposure. Lead poisoning concerns environmental health, even if it is not immediately infectious. Safeguarding other animals involves preventing entry into contaminated areas and properly disposing of objects that contain lead.

Equine

Immune-Mediated: Equine Recurrent Uveitis (Moon Blindness).

Horses are primarily affected by equine recurrent uveitis, also known as moon blindness. An inflammatory response inflames the uveal tract (Zisopoulou et al., 2023). Although uncommon in species other than horses, this condition causes recurrent episodes of ocular inflammation, which can lead to blindness or impaired vision. Clinical symptoms include hearing, corneal oedema, photophobia, and ocular discomfort. Ocular ultrasonography, ophthalmic examination, and serological testing are all part of the diagnostic process.

Anti-inflammatory drugs, topical treatments, and addressing underlying reasons are all part of the treatment; the prognosis varies based on the severity of the problem and the patient's response to treatment. Although no specific vaccination is available, preventive measures include genetic selection, insect control, and environmental management (Gilger et al., 2004). Equine recurrent uveitis is not zoonotic, and controlling its spread necessitates isolating affected horses, maintaining proper hygiene in stables, and implementing screening protocols for new arrivals to prevent the introduction of infectious agents causing uveitis.

Congenital/Genetic: Cleft Palate

A gap in the roof of the mouth results from the inadequate fusion of the palatal shelves during embryonic development, which causes cleft palate, a congenital/genetic abnormality. Although canines are typically affected, other species may also be impacted by this illness. Cleft palates in dogs can cause serious problems, including nursing, an elevated risk of aspiration pneumonia, malnourishment, and respiratory discomfort (Roman et al., 2019). The mentioned viral infection can also induce similar clinical difficulties in horses, ruminants, and cats, albeit these are less prevalent. Puppies affected may exhibit coughing, choking, nasal discharge, and failure to thrive, often accompanied by malnourishment and respiratory infections. In addition to the fundamental methods of diagnosis, such as physical examination and oral inspection, radiography is utilised to ascertain the extent of the abnormality.

The main course of treatment is surgical correction; the procedure's outcome depends on the extent of the deformity and its degree of rectification. Genetic screening and avoiding pairings with people who have a history of cleft palate are two responsible breeding practices that are part of prevention methods. Genetic control is the mainstay of preventative interventions because no specific vaccine exists. There are no concerns about the contagious spread of cleft palate because it is not zoonotic, meaning it cannot be transmitted from animals to humans (Roman et al., 2019). To manage and minimise the effects of cleft palate in veterinary medicine, a thorough strategy that includes early diagnosis, suitable surgical intervention, and preventive measures in breeding techniques is necessary.

Ruminant or Swine

Giardia

The leading cause of Giardia, which is extremely dangerous to the health of ruminants and pigs, is the protozoan parasite Giardia duodenalis. People, dogs, cats, cattle, sheep, and goats are among the many species afflicted by the parasite. In ruminants and swine, Giardia infections commonly result in diarrhoea, weight loss, and decreased growth rates, all of which reduce total herd productivity (Adam, 2021). Afflicted animals may exhibit sporadic or chronic diarrhoea, weight loss, dehydration, and poor physical condition. Typically, faecal testing for Giardia cysts or trophozoites employs microscopy or antigen detection assays, such as ELISA, to confirm the diagnosis.

Antiprotozoal drugs, such as metronidazole or fenbendazole, are administered as part of the treatment; a good prognosis is anticipated with early intervention. The primary goals of preventive measures are to minimise environmental contamination, maintain clean animal housing facilities, and prevent overcrowding (Adam, 2021). Humans can contract the zoonotic disease Giardia by entering faecal-oral contact with sick animals. Giardia transmission within animal populations can only be prevented by maintaining clean water sources and adopting effective hygiene practices.

Eimeria Spp

Eimeria spp., protozoan parasites that cause coccidiosis, predominantly affect ruminants, including cattle, sheep, goats, and swine. Unlike Giardia, Eimeria infections are specific to livestock and do not commonly affect other species (Ayana et al., 2022). Enteritis, diarrhoea, dehydration, weight loss, and a reduction in feed conversion efficiency are all consequences of infections in ruminants and pigs, which cause significant financial losses in livestock production. Clinical signs include bloody or watery diarrhoea, dehydration, lethargy, and reduced feed intake. Molecular or microscopic methods are used to diagnose Eimeria oocysts in faeces.

Treatment involves administering anticoccidial drugs, such as sulfonamides or ionophores, with the prognosis contingent on the severity of the infection and the timeliness of treatment. Changing the grazing area, utilising anticoccidial drugs, and maintaining cleanliness are a few examples of prevention techniques. For particular cattle species, vaccines against Eimeria spp. are available, protecting against specific parasite types (Ayana et al., 2022). Eimeria infections in cattle are not zoonotic, unlike Giardia infections, and controlling the infectious spread requires avoiding overcrowding, maintaining good hygiene, and implementing biosecurity procedures.

Exotics (can include avian, amphibian, reptile, or pocket pets)

Metabolic: Scurvy

In exotic pets, such as guinea pigs, monkeys, and some bird species like parrots, a vitamin C shortage causes scurvy. Vitamin C is necessary for the production of collagen. Scurvy in guinea pigs manifests as poor nutrition, swollen joints, bleeding, sluggish wound healing, and a rough coat (Keeble, 2023). Scurvy-prone monkeys and birds, particularly parrots, also have similar clinical symptoms. Among the symptoms are lameness, swollen and bleeding gums, and subcutaneous haemorrhage. Clinical symptoms, medical history, and blood tests are used to detect vitamin C levels and make the diagnosis. Treatment typically involves oral or injectable vitamin C supplementation, offering a favourable prognosis with prompt intervention.

On the other hand, untreated situations could cause permanent harm (Keeble, 2023). A diet high in vitamin C and fresh produce is one preventive method. There is no vaccine to prevent scurvy or to prevent the risk of zoonotic transfer or infectious dissemination.

Neoplastic: Melanoma.

One type of neoplastic cancer that is frequently brought on by genetic flaws is melanoma. Melanocytes are responsible for the colour of mucous membranes and skin. Numerous exotic creatures, such as chameleons and frogs, are among the many that it can injure. Melanoma in chameleons typically manifests as pigmented skin lesions or masses, which can lead to subsequent infections and local tissue loss (Smith et al., 2002). While less common, frogs may also develop melanoma, showing similar clinical signs. These signs include alterations in skin colour, ulceration, bleeding, swelling, and lameness if internal organs are involved. Biopsy samples from suspected lesions are examined histopathologically to provide a diagnosis.

Treatment options may include surgical excision, chemotherapy, or radiation therapy, depending on tumour characteristics and metastasis, with prognosis varying accordingly. Preventive methods, such as skin monitoring and routine veterinary checks, aid in early detection and treatment (Smith et al., 2002). Vaccination is not applicable for melanoma, as infectious agents do not cause it, and it is not zoonotic, meaning it poses no risk of transmission between animals and humans. Additionally, melanoma is not contagious and does not spread from one animal to another.

Conclusion

To summarise, innovative techniques are crucial for diagnosing, treating, and preventing a wide range of diseases that affect various animal species and are addressed by veterinary medicine. A thorough study examines the challenges of treating animal illnesses such as rabies and scurvy. Veterinary environments place a strong emphasis on the value of informed techniques, meticulous diligence, prevention, treatment options, and zoonotic dangers.

References

Adam, R. D. (2021). Giardia duodenalis: biology and pathogenesis. *Clinical microbiology reviews, 34(4),* e00024- 19. https://pubmed.ncbi.nlm.nih.gov/34378955/

Altınok-Yipel, F., Yipel, M., & Tekeli, İ. O. (2022). Health risk assessment of essential and toxic metals in canned/pouched food on kitten and adult cats: An animal health risk assessment adaptation assay. *Biological Trace Element Research, 200(4),* 1937-1948. https://pubmed.ncbi.nlm.nih.gov/34432269/

Astuty, A. T. J. E., Tjahajati, I., & Nugroho, W. S. (2020). Detection of feline idiopathic cystitis as the cause of feline lower urinary tract disease in Sleman Regency, Indonesia. *Veterinary World, 13(6),* 1108. https://www.veterinaryworld.org/Vol.13/June-2020/13.pdf

Ayana, D., Temesgen, K., Kumsa, B., & Alkadir, G. (2022). Dry season Eimeria infection in dairy cattle and sheep in and around Adama and Bishoftu Towns, Oromia, Ethiopia. Veterinary Medicine: Research and Reports, 235-245. https://www.ncbi.nlm.nih.gov/pmc/articles/PMC9470120/

Gilger, B. C., & Michau, T. M. (2004). Equine recurrent uveitis: new methods of management. *Veterinary Clinics: Equine Practice, 20(2),* 417–427. https://pubmed.ncbi.nlm.nih.gov/15271431/

Keeble, E. (2023). Guinea pig nutrition: what do we know? In Practice, 45(4), 200–210. https://www.research.ed.ac.uk/en/publications/clinical-review-guinea-pig-nutrition-what-do-we-know

Nivy, R., Segev, G., Rimer, D., Bruchim, Y., Aroch, I., & Mazaki-Tovi, M. (2019). A prospective randomised study of the efficacy of 2 treatment protocols in preventing the recurrence of clinical signs in 51 male cats with obstructive idiopathic cystitis. *Journal of Veterinary Internal Medicine, 33(5),* 2117-2123. https://onlinelibrary.wiley.com/doi/full/10.1111/jvim.15594

O'Brien, N. S., Hatke, A. L., Camire, A. C., & Marconi, R. T. (2021). Human and Veterinary Vaccines for Lyme Disease. *Current Issues in Molecular Biology, 42(1),* 191–222. https://pubmed.ncbi.nlm.nih.gov/33289681/

Roman, N., Carney, P. C., Fiani, N., & Peralta, S. (2019). Incidence patterns of orofacial clefts in purebred dogs. *PLS One, 14(11),* e0224574. https://journals.plos.org/plosone/article?id=10.1371/journal.pone.0224574

Rupprecht, C., Kuzmin, I., & Meslin, F. (2017). Lyssaviruses and rabies: current problems, concerns, contradictions, and controversies. *F1000Research, 6.* https://f1000research.com/articles/6-184

Smith, S. H., Goldschmidt, M. H., & McManus, P. M. (2002). A comparative review of melanocytic neoplasms. *Veterinary Pathology, 39(6),* 651–678. https://journals.sagepub.com/doi/pdf/10.1354/vp.39-6-651

Stoewen, D. L., Coe, J. B., MacMartin, C., Stone, E. A., & Dewey, C. E. (2019). Identification of illness uncertainty in veterinary oncology: implications for service. *Frontiers in Veterinary Science, 6,* 147. https://www.frontiersin.org/articles/10.3389/fvets.2019.00147/full

World Health Organisation. (2019, September 28). World Rabies Day 2019. https://www.who.int/news/item/28-09-2019-united-against-rabies-collaboration-celebrates-one-year-of-progress-towards-zero-human-rabies-deaths-by-2030

Zisopoulou, A. M., Vyhnalová, N., Jánová, E., Kološ, F., & Krisová, Š. (2023). The correlation between the intraocular pressure, central corneal thickness, and signalment of the horse. *Acta Veterinaria Brno, 92(3),* 271-278. https://actavet.vfu.cz/92/3/0271/

Chapter 2

An investigation into drug side effects (Vancomycin)

Content

An investigation into drug side effects (Vancomycin)

Gram-positive infections caused by bacteria that can be dangerous undergo therapy with glycopeptide antibiotics, such as Vancomycin. It is helpful in the fight against illnesses caused by penicillin-sensitive bacteria and methicillin-resistant Staphylococcus aureus (MRSA). Vancomycin is occasionally used off-label when the primary preventive fails to cure severe Clostridium difficile infections (Hasmukharay et al., 2023). It is critical to recognise adverse drug reactions (ADRs) and medication mistakes or errors associated with them because Vancomycin has a narrow therapeutic window and the ability to cause serious side effects. By emphasising this comprehension analysis, healthcare providers must ensure that patients are safe and that treatment outcomes are accurate.

Adverse Effects and Medication Error Statistics

Common adverse effects associated with Vancomycin that may be severe and prolonged include ototoxicity and nephrotoxicity. Nephrotoxicity can affect 5–43% of Vancomycin users, depending on therapy duration and dosage, as reported by Rybak et al. (2020).

Despite its lack of prevalence, up to 10% of patients may experience ototoxicity, especially in situations involving prolonged use and high serum levels.
An unusual adverse effect is "red man syndrome," which manifests as flushing, dermatitis, and hypotension brought on by the drug's fast infusion. Up to 50% of patients may experience complications if the infusion rate is not controlled. Although rare, serious adverse effects such as anaphylaxis, thrombocytopenia, and neutropenia are possible.
Prescription errors are more likely to occur when using Vancomycin due to its complex dosing requirements, which necessitate close monitoring of serum levels. Typical mistakes include administering the wrong dosage, failing to adjust doses according to renal function, and using incorrect infusion rates, which can result in infusion-related adverse responses. A study by Naseralallah et al. (2020) found that nearly 20% of vancomycin prescriptions contained dose errors, underscoring the importance of cautious administration and close monitoring.

Preventive measures and nursing interventions

Vancomycin medication errors and adverse drug reactions can be prevented by following preventive measures that include patient education, dosing

procedures, and monitoring. Important tactics consist of the monitoring of therapeutic drugs (TDM). Regularly monitoring the serum level of Vancomycin is essential. TDM assists in dose modification to minimise toxicity and maintain therapeutic levels. Levels must be examined before the fourth dosage to guarantee steady-state concentration (Al-Sulaiti et al., 2019). Regulation of infusion rates is the second strategy. To prevent red man syndrome, Vancomycin should be administered gradually, typically over a minimum of 60 minutes. Hasmukharay et al. (2023) suggest extending the infusion period to 90-120 minutes when administering greater doses.
Dosing guidelines and uniformity make up the third strategy. Medication errors are reduced when consistent dosing protocols and standards are followed, including dose modifications for specific patient populations (such as pediatric, elderly, or those with renal impairment). Finally, patient education is a tactic. Adverse drug responses (ADRs) can appear as symptoms of an allergic reaction, unusual bleeding, or hearing loss. Patients need to be made aware of these warning signs. Patients need to notify their doctor of these symptoms as soon as possible.

Utilising nursing interventions is crucial for implementing these preventive measures. Healthcare professionals should ensure proper medication administration and adhere to recommended infusion rates, which is primarily the responsibility of nurses. They also perform regular evaluations of renal function and promptly schedule TDM. Nurses also educate patients about potential adverse effects and the importance of keeping follow-up appointments to monitor their progress. They also guarantee that the medical staff communicates clearly to quickly address differences in the patient's reaction to the medication.

Diagnosis for Handling Adverse Reactions and Side Effects

The following diagnostic procedures are crucial for tracking and managing vancomycin-related side effects and adverse reactions.

- Blood urea nitrogen and serum creatinine (BUN) are frequently observed. These parameters facilitate the early detection of nephrotoxic symptoms. Elevated levels necessitate dose modification, as they indicate compromised renal function (Rybak et al., 2020).
- Vancomycin Peak Amounts. To ensure that therapeutic levels are maintained without reaching

dangerous concentrations, trough levels should be evaluated before the next dose, preferably after the third or fourth dose (Naseralallah et al., 2020).

- They are testing for audiometry. Baseline and recurrent hearing tests are recommended for patients undergoing prolonged vancomycin therapy, particularly those receiving higher doses or concurrent ototoxic medications.
- Total Blood Count (TCB). Frequent CBCs aid in detecting thrombocytopenia and neutropenia, two haematological side effects. Any notable modifications require additional research and may necessitate stopping the medication.
- Panel Electrolyte. Vancomycin can lead to imbalances, especially hypokalemia, which might worsen the patient's state. Hence, it is imperative to monitor electrolytes.

Evidence supporting the function of these diagnostics in the early identification and treatment of ADRs related to Vancomycin is provided. For example, Hasmukharay et al.'s thorough 2023 study highlights the importance of routinely checking vancomycin and serum creatinine levels to prevent renal impairment and ensure appropriate dosing.

Conclusion

In summary, although there are considerable risks of adverse effects and prescription errors associated with the use of Vancomycin, it remains an essential antibiotic for treating severe Gram-positive infections. Healthcare practitioners can mitigate these hazards by implementing preventive measures, such as therapeutic medication monitoring, appropriate dosage adjustments, controlled infusion rates, and thorough patient education. A crucial component of successfully implementing these methods is the application of practical nursing interventions. Frequent diagnostic testing is necessary to ensure patient safety and optimal treatment outcomes, as it enables the prompt detection and management of side effects.

References

Al-Sulaiti, F. K., Nader, A. M., Saad, M. O., Shaukat, A., Parakadavathu, R., Elzubair, A., ... & Awaisu, A. (2019). Clinical and pharmacokinetic outcomes of peak-trough-based versus trough-based vancomycin therapeutic drug monitoring approaches: A pragmatic randomised controlled trial. *European Journal of Drug Metabolism and Pharmacokinetics, 44,* 639–652. https://pubmed.ncbi.nlm.nih.gov/30919233/

Hasmukharay, K., Ngoi, S. T., Saedon, N. I., Tan, K. M., Khor, H. M., Chin, A. V., ... & Ponnampalavanar, S. S. L. S. (2023). Evaluation of methicillin-resistant Staphylococcus aureus (MRSA) bacteremia: Epidemiology, clinical characteristics, and outcomes in the older patients in a tertiary teaching hospital in Malaysia. *BMC infectious diseases, 23(1),* 241. https://www.ncbi.nlm.nih.gov/pmc/articles/PMC10111773/

Naseralallah, L. M., Hussain, T. A., Jaam, M., & Pawluk, S. A. (2020). The impact of pharmacist interventions on medication errors in hospitalised pediatric patients is a systematic review and meta-analysis. *International Journal of Clinical Pharmacy, 42(4),* 979–994. https://doi.org/10.1007/s11096-020-01034-z

Rybak, M. J., Le, J., Lodise, T. P., Levine, D. P., Bradley, J. S., Liu, C., ... & Lomaestro, B. M. (2020). Therapeutic monitoring of Vancomycin for serious methicillin-resistant Staphylococcus aureus infections: a revised consensus guideline and review by the American Society of Health-System Pharmacists, the Infectious Diseases Society of America, the Pediatric Infectious Diseases Society, and the Society of Infectious Diseases Pharmacists. *American Journal of Health-System Pharmacy, 77(11),* 835–864. https://pubmed.ncbi.nlm.nih.gov/32658968/

Chapter 3

An Overview of Research Ethics Practices

Content

An Overview of Research Ethics Practices

Abstract.

They treat research participants with respect and protect their well-being. It is essential to ensure the trustworthiness and accuracy of scientific studies. In this paper, we will examine two primary types of research: qualitative research, which employs stories from individuals to gain an understanding of phenomena, and quantitative research, which utilises numbers and statistical analysis. The outlined steps include formulating research questions and hypotheses, evaluating the body of Literature, sampling, techniques, and presenting results. The document provides detailed information to guarantee that participants are appropriately informed about the study and their rights. It also covers the principles and procedures for obtaining informed consent. Furthermore, it discusses unethical research practices, including data fabrication, plagiarism, and failure to obtain informed consent. This analysis emphasises the significance of following ethical principles, drawing on findings from Nowak and Colsch. Brown's Evidence-Based Nursing emphasises the connection between research and practice. Such adherence highlights the vital role that ethical norms play in conducting responsible research, thereby improving the quality of research outputs. Additionally, it fosters confidence in the scientific community and safeguards the well-being of participants.

Keywords: Ethical research procedures, informed consent, unethical research process.

Overview of the Types of Research.

Typically, there are two primary classifications of research: qualitative and quantitative. Investigating phenomena through detailed narrative descriptions is the primary objective of qualitative research. Focus groups, interviews, and ethnography are among the methods commonly employed to understand the underlying assumptions, motivations, and causes of a phenomenon (Mirza et al., 2023). This type of research provides profound insights into complex topics by analysing non-numerical data. In contrast, quantitative research attempts to generate numerical data or transform data into useful statistics. The mentioned approach is used to quantify the problem. Researchers use systematic techniques to test theories and examine correlations between variables. These techniques include surveys, experiments, and observational studies. Quantitative research uses statistical analysis to identify trends and facts that are generally used.

Components Involved in Conducting Research.

Several key elements comprise the research process. They all play a part in the ultimate success and integrity of the study. The first component is the Research Question. The research question determines the study's focus. It must be time-bound, relevant, quantifiable, achievable, and specific (SMART). The second component is a hypothesis. It is a verifiable claim that forecasts the anticipated result of the research. It gives the research a direction (Nowak & Colsch, 2024). The third one is a review of the Literature. It involves a comprehensive review of past studies and theoretical perspectives on the topic of interest. The process provides a framework for assessing current findings and identifying areas where knowledge gaps exist.

The fourth component is sampling. It involves selecting a subset of the population to participate in a study. Based on the objectives and study design, the study can be conducted either stratified or randomly. The fifth one is methods. The steps and strategies for gathering and analysing data are described in this section. It explains the tools, data collection procedures, and study design. The last element is findings. The outcomes of the data analysis are known as findings. Insights into the research topic and evidence for or against the hypothesis should be provided clearly and methodically.

Getting Informed Consent to Take Part in Research.

An essential ethical prerequisite for any study involving human subjects is the principle of informed consent. It guarantees that people are completely informed about the requirements before consenting to participate. During this phase, potential volunteers are provided with thorough information on the study's goals, design, methods, risks, benefits, and their rights as participants (Wu et al., 2024). This typically begins with a pamphlet or information sheet that provides a clear and concise explanation of the study. This paper describes the research methodology, participant expectations, and the use and protection of the participants' data.

After reading this information, people are encouraged to ask questions and receive straightforward, truthful responses to inform their decision-making. Researchers must emphasise that participation is entirely voluntary and that individuals are free to leave at any time without incurring any fees or forfeiting any benefits. This promise guarantees ethical integrity and fosters trust. Participants' consent is officially recorded, typically through a signed consent form, after they have reviewed all the study details and decided to participate. This signed paper is essential to conducting ethical research and recording the voluntary agreement.

Unethical Research Practices.

Credibility and integrity in research are closely tied to ethical considerations. Misconduct in research can take many different forms, such as fabricating evidence to justify incorrect conclusions, which is one type of falsification, among other types of misconduct. The following action is plagiarism. It is repeating someone else's ideas without giving credit (Sivasubramaniam et al., 2021). Another unethical action is failing to obtain informed consent. There is a need for more information about the study participants or to obtain their permission. Next is fraud. They are providing participants with false information about the study's purpose. Another concern is the potential harm to participants, which is placing them at risk without adequate physical or mental protection. The last one is a private violation, which involves neglecting to preserve the privacy and confidentiality of participant data.

References

Mirza, H., Mirza, C., & Bellalem, F. (2023). Ethical considerations in qualitative research: Summary guidelines for novice social science researchers. *Social Studies and Research Journal, 11(1),* 441-449. https://www.researchgate.net/publication/370838199_Ethical_Considerations_in_Qualitative_Research_Summary_Guidelines_for_Novice_Social_Science_Researchers

Nowak, E. W., & Colsch, R. (2024). Brown's Evidence-based nursing: The research-practice connection (5th ed.). *Jones & Bartlett Learning, LLC.* https://www.jblearning.com/catalog/productdetails/9781284275889

Sivasubramaniam, S. D., Cosentino, M., Ribeiro, L., & Marino, F. (2021). Unethical practices within medical research and publication–An exploratory study. *International Journal for Educational Integrity, 17,* 1–13. https://edintegrity.biomedcentral.com/articles/10.1007/s40979-021-00072-y

Wu, C., Wang, N., Wang, Q., Wang, C., Wei, Z., Wu, Z., ... & Jiang, X. (2024). Participants' understanding of informed consent in clinical trials: A systematic review and updated meta-analysis. *Plos one, 19(1),*

e0295784. https://doi.org/10.1371/journal.
pone.0295784

Chapter 4

Importance of Carrying Around Devices to Reduce Cybersecurity Risks in Healthcare.

Content

4. Discuss the advantages and risks of using portable devices in healthcare.

5. Explain how the five steps of the cybersecurity framework (from the textbook) apply to using portable devices and help manage risk.

6. Overall, do you agree or disagree with using portable devices in healthcare? Why or why not?

References

Importance of Carrying Around Devices to Reduce Cybersecurity Risks in Healthcare

The increasing use of portable devices in healthcare, including smartphones, tablets, and wearable technology, has significantly transformed patient care by enhancing accessibility, communication, and facilitating real-time data sharing. These tools enable healthcare professionals to remotely monitor patients, access medical records instantly, and provide timely interventions, ultimately enhancing the efficiency and quality of care. However, alongside these technological advancements come notable concerns related to data privacy and cybersecurity. As highlighted by Syafrizal et al. (2020), the widespread use of portable devices introduces vulnerabilities that may compromise sensitive patient information if not properly managed. This journal critically examines the advantages and limitations of using portable devices in healthcare settings. It also evaluates the effectiveness of current cybersecurity protocols in mitigating potential risks. Through an objective analysis, the journal assesses the overall contribution of portable technology to the healthcare sector while emphasising the importance of maintaining secure, ethical, and patient-centred practices.

Discuss the advantages and risks of using portable devices in healthcare.

Integrating portable devices into healthcare delivery has transformed how medical professionals access, manage, and utilise patient data. With the ability to retrieve critical health information at any time and from virtually any location, these devices empower healthcare providers to make timely and well-informed clinical decisions right at the point of care (Syafrizal et al., 2022). Whether in hospitals, clinics, or even remote or home-based settings, the portability and connectivity of modern digital tools eliminate many of the traditional barriers associated with data retrieval and decision-making. This improves patient outcomes, faster diagnosis, and more accurate treatment interventions.

Mobile health applications play a pivotal role in this technological evolution. These apps are not merely passive tools for documentation; they actively contribute to improved care coordination, remote patient monitoring, and enhanced communication between patients and providers. Through secure and user-friendly interfaces, mobile apps enable continuous monitoring of vital signs, medication adherence, and the management of chronic diseases.

For example, a patient with diabetes can use a mobile app to log blood sugar levels, which are then instantly accessible to their care team. This allows for real-time feedback and adjustments to the treatment plan, potentially preventing complications and hospitalisation.

Moreover, these apps facilitate seamless communication across interdisciplinary teams. Nurses, physicians, specialists, and support staff can collaborate more efficiently when patient information, test results, and treatment updates are available via portable devices. This real-time information exchange reduces errors, eliminates redundant testing, and shortens response times. Consequently, healthcare providers can deliver more coordinated and patient-centred care, fostering better health outcomes and greater patient satisfaction.

Remote patient monitoring (RPM) is another significant advantage of portable devices and mobile apps. RPM enables clinicians to remotely track patient health data, often from the patient's home. This capability is especially vital for managing chronic conditions such as hypertension, heart failure, and COPD. With wearable sensors and mobile interfaces, patient data, including heart rate, oxygen saturation, and physical activity, can be transmitted continuously to healthcare providers. Not only does this reduce the need for frequent office visits, but it also enables the early detection of potential health issues, allowing for proactive interventions.

Security and privacy are paramount when using portable devices in healthcare. These devices are increasingly equipped with encryption protocols, multi-factor authentication, and other cybersecurity measures to protect sensitive patient information. This is essential for compliance with healthcare regulations, such as HIPAA, and for maintaining patient trust. When used for secure internal communication among staff, these devices can replace outdated systems, such as pagers and insecure messaging platforms, providing a safer and more efficient alternative for clinical communication.

Access to electronic health records (EHRs) via portable devices is another significant factor in improving healthcare workflow and productivity (Syafrizal et al., 2022). With mobile access to EHRs, clinicians can review patient histories, lab results, imaging, and medication lists during rounds, in emergency scenarios, or even when consulting from outside the hospital. This streamlined access facilitates faster clinical decision-making and reduces administrative burdens, enabling providers to focus more on patient care.

However, the convenience of portable devices comes at a cost. These devices' inherent susceptibility to theft, loss, and malware infection poses a serious threat to patient data confidentiality. Weak passwords, insufficient device encryption, and insecure Wi-Fi networks can initiate cyberattacks that compromise patient privacy and result in data breaches. Sharing these devices is, therefore, more convenient, but it also raises the possibility of unintentional data leaks, especially in hospital settings where staff members lack the necessary education and training.

Explain how the five steps of the cybersecurity framework (from the textbook) apply to using portable devices and help manage risk.

The five phases of the NIST Cybersecurity Framework provide a comprehensive and structured approach for managing cybersecurity risks associated with using portable devices in healthcare settings. This framework is especially valuable given the growing reliance on mobile technologies to improve communication, patient monitoring, and data accessibility. The first phase is Identify, where healthcare organisations must develop an accurate inventory of all portable devices that connect to their network. This includes smartphones, tablets, laptops, and wearable medical technologies. Identifying these assets also involves recognising potential vulnerabilities and understanding how each device interacts with sensitive patient data and critical systems. Understanding the organisation's digital environment is the foundation for all subsequent risk management strategies.

The second phase is Protect, which focuses on implementing safeguards to limit or contain the impact of potential cybersecurity events. According to Sean (2015), it is vital to encrypt all sensitive data both at rest and during transmission to prevent unauthorised access. Enforcing strong password policies, utilising biometric authentication, and turning off unnecessary features such as Bluetooth or location services can significantly reduce exposure to threats. In addition, Mobile Device Management (MDM) systems offer centralised oversight of device security. These systems allow IT administrators to configure security settings, manage app usage, and, importantly, remotely wipe lost, stolen, or compromised devices.

The Identify and Protect phases lay the groundwork for a secure mobile technology environment in healthcare. When executed correctly, they help safeguard patient information, support regulatory compliance, and ensure that the benefits of mobile devices, such as improved efficiency, communication, and access to care, are realised without compromising cybersecurity. These proactive measures also build a strong culture of accountability and data protection among staff, ultimately strengthening institutional resilience in an increasingly digital healthcare landscape.

The third is Detect. Monitoring device logs and network activity to spot unusual activities is essential. By implementing endpoint security solutions and intrusion detection systems (IDS), it is feasible to identify potential breaches, and unauthorised access attempts can be identified. The fourth step is to respond. A well-defined incident response plan ensures a swift and coordinated response to cyberattacks. Healthcare institutions must establish procedures for identifying compromised devices, halting the security breach, contacting the affected parties, and investigating the root cause (Sean, 2015). Regular training for staff in reporting suspicious activities and following cybersecurity protocols is vital. Recovering is the fifth step. Having a cyber resilience plan in place allows for quicker recovery from a cyberattack. Backups of critical data stored on portable devices ensure swift restoration in case of data loss or device malfunction. Disaster recovery plans should consider scenarios involving mobile device compromise and outline steps for resuming normal operations efficiently.

Overall, do you agree or disagree with the use of portable devices in healthcare? Why or why not?

I strongly advocate for integrating portable electronic devices into healthcare, provided that robust security measures are established and maintained. These technologies significantly benefit clinical practice, notably enhancing the communication, coordination, and efficiency of healthcare teams. According to Maryville University (2021), mobile devices such as smartphones, tablets, and wearable health monitors streamline workflows, reduce delays in care, and enable real-time data sharing. This leads to quicker decision-making, improved diagnostics, and better patient outcomes. Moreover, portable devices support telehealth and remote monitoring, making healthcare more accessible, especially for patients in rural or underserved areas.

However, integrating such technology must be approached with a strong emphasis on security. Protecting patient health information is a legal obligation under frameworks like HIPAA and an ethical imperative. Healthcare organisations should adopt comprehensive cybersecurity strategies, such as those outlined in the NIST Cybersecurity Framework. This includes identifying and managing risks, protecting systems and data, detecting threats, responding effectively to incidents, and recovering from breaches.

In addition to technical safeguards, fostering a culture of cybersecurity awareness among all healthcare staff is crucial. Regular training and policy updates ensure employees understand how to handle devices responsibly and recognise potential threats such as phishing attacks or unsecured networks. By striking a balance between technological innovation and stringent security protocols, healthcare institutions can fully leverage the advantages of portable devices. This approach not only improves the quality and efficiency of care but also reinforces patient trust, safeguards sensitive information, and upholds the integrity of the healthcare system.

References

Syafrizal, M., Selamat, S. R., & Zakaria, N. A. (2020). Analysis of cybersecurity standard and framework components. International Journal of Communication Networks and Information Security, 12(3), 417-432. https://www.ijcnis.org/index.php/ijcnis/article/view/4817

Sean P. Murphy. (2015, January 15). *Healthcare Information Security and Privacy*. McGraw-Hill. https://www.amazon.com/Healthcare-Information-Security-Privacy-Murphy/dp/0071831797

Maryville University. (2021, November 2). Mobile Technology in Healthcare: Trends and Benefits. https://online.maryville.edu/blog/mobile-technology-in-healthcare/

Chapter 5

Addison Disease

Content

- Drugs

Etomidate,

- Haemorrhage into Adrenal Glands

Clinical Manifestations

Laboratory Findings

Differential Diagnosis

Treatment

Introduction

Addison Disease

- Addison's disease (or Addison's disease) is adrenocortical insufficiency due to the destruction or dysfunction of the entire adrenal cortex.
- It affects glucocorticoid and mineralocorticoid function.
- The disease onset usually occurs when 90% or more of both adrenal cortices are dysfunctional or destroyed.

anatomy

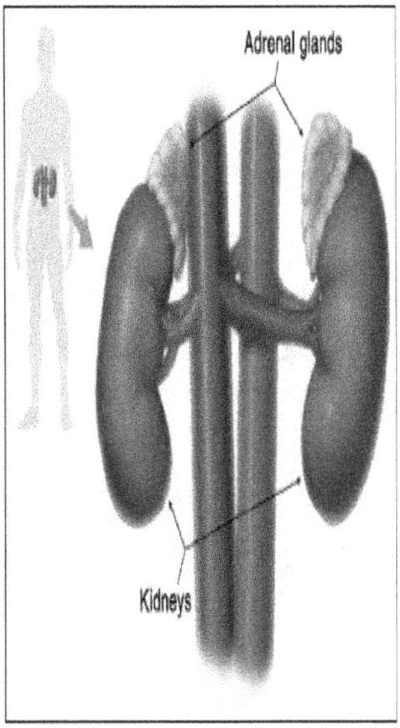

•

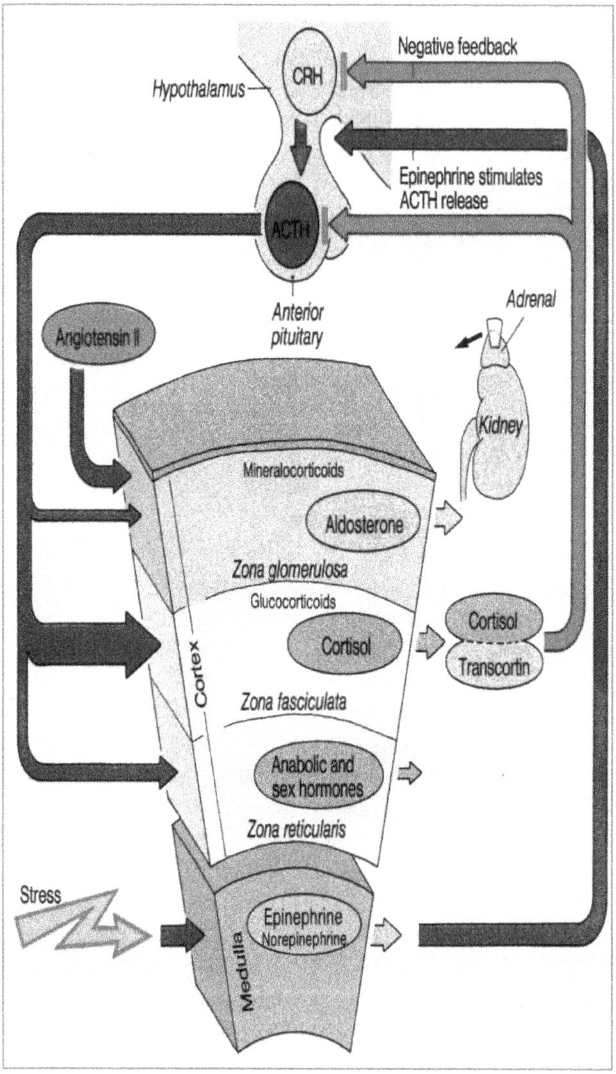

• Patients usually present with features of both glucocorticoid and mineralocorticoid deficiency.

- The predominant symptoms vary depending on the duration of the disease.
- Patients may present with clinical features of chronic Addison's disease or in acute Addisonian crisis precipitated by stress factors such as infection, trauma, surgery, vomiting, diarrhoea, or noncompliance with replacement steroids.

Primary Adrenal Insufficiency

- Primary adrenal insufficiency in children is most frequently caused by genetic conditions that are often but not always manifested in infancy and less often by acquired problems such as autoimmune conditions.
- Susceptibility to autoimmune conditions often has a genetic basis, so these distinctions are not absolute.

Inherited Etiologies

- **Inborn Defects of Steroid Synthesis**

- The most common causes of adrenocortical insufficiency in infancy are the salt-losing forms of congenital adrenal hyperplasia.
- Approximately 75% of infants with 21-hydroxylase deficiency, almost all infants with lipoid

adrenal hyperplasia, and most infants with a deficiency of 3β 3β-hydroxysteroid dehydrogenase manifest salt-losing symptoms in the newborn period because they are unable to synthesise either cortisol or aldosterone.

Adrenal Hypoplasia Congenita

- Adrenal hypoplasia congenita (AHC) is a relatively frequent cause of adrenal failure in males, along with congenital adrenal hyperplasia, autoimmune disease, and adrenoleukodystrophy (ALD).
- AHC is predominantly a failure of development of the definitive zone of the adrenal cortex; the fetal zone may be relatively normal.
- Adrenal insufficiency generally becomes evident as the fetal zone involutes postnatally, with an onset in infancy or the first two years of life, but occasionally in later childhood or adulthood.
- In some cases, aldosterone deficiency becomes evident before cortisol deficiency.
- The disorder is caused by a mutation of the *DAX1 (NR0B1)* gene, a nuclear hormone receptor family member, located on Xp21. Males with AHC often do not undergo puberty, owing to

hypogonadotropic hypogonadism caused by the same mutated *DAX1* gene.

- **Cryptorchidism,**

Sometimes noted in these males is probably an early manifestation of hypogonadotropic hypogonadism, but often testicular function in infants is standard, with a typical or even an unusually prolonged testosterone surge in the first month of life.

- AHC occasionally occurs as part of a *contiguous gene deletion* syndrome together with Duchenne muscular dystrophy, glycerol kinase deficiency, cognitive impairment, or a combination of these conditions.

Other Genetic Causes of Adrenal Hypoplasia

- The transcription factor SF-1 is required for adrenal and gonadal development
- Males with a heterozygous mutation in SF-1 *(NR5A1)* have impaired development of the testes despite the presence of a normal copy of the gene on the other chromosome. They can appear to

be female, similar to patients with lipoid adrenal hyperplasia.

- Rarely, such patients also have adrenal insufficiency.
- Adrenal hypoplasia is also occasionally seen in patients with Pallister-Hall syndrome caused by mutations in the GLI3 oncogene.

Adrenoleukodystrophy

- In ALD, adrenocortical deficiency is associated with demyelination in the central nervous system.
- High levels of long-chain fatty acids are found in tissues and body fluids, resulting from impaired β-oxidation in the peroxisomes.
- The most common form of ALD is an X-linked disorder with various presentations.

- The most common clinical picture is of a degenerative neurologic disorder appearing in childhood or adolescence and progressing to severe dementia and deterioration of vision, hearing, speech, and gait, with death occurring within a few years.
- Neurologic symptoms may be subtle at onset, sometimes consisting only of behavioural changes or deteriorating academic performance.

- Generalised but incomplete alopecia, resembling that of chemotherapy, is a characteristic but inconsistent finding.
- A milder form of X-linked ALD is Adrenomyeloneuropathy, which begins in later adolescence or early adulthood.
- Patients may have evidence of adrenal insufficiency before, at the time of, or after neurologic symptoms develop, often with years separating their presentation.
- X-linked ALD is caused by mutations in the *ABCD1* gene located on Xq28.
- The gene encodes a transmembrane transporter involved in importing very-long-chain fatty acids into peroxisomes.
- There is no correlation between the degree of neurologic impairment and the severity of adrenal insufficiency.
- Prenatal diagnosis by DNA analysis, family screening by very-long-chain fatty acid assays, and mutation analysis are available. Women who are heterozygous carriers of the X-linked ALD gene can develop symptoms in midlife or later; adrenal insufficiency is a rare occurrence.
- Neonatal ALD is a rare autosomal recessive disorder. Infants have neurologic

deterioration and have or acquire evidence of adrenocortical dysfunction.

- Most patients have severe, progressive cognitive impairment and die before 5 years of age.
- This disorder is a subset of Zellweger (cerebrohepatorenal) syndrome, in which peroxisomes do not develop at all owing to mutations in any of several genes (*PEX5, PEX1, PEX10, PEX13,* and *PEX26*) controlling the development of this organelle.

Familial Glucocorticoid Deficiency

- A form of chronic adrenal insufficiency characterised by isolated deficiency of glucocorticoids, elevated levels of ACTH, and generally normal aldosterone production, although salt-losing manifestations, as are present in most other forms of adrenal insufficiency, occasionally occur.
- Patients mainly have hypoglycemia, seizures, and increased pigmentation during the first decade of life.
- Affects both sexes equally and is inherited in an autosomal recessive manner.
- There is marked adrenocortical atrophy with relative sparing of the zona glomerulosa.

- Mutations in the gene for the ACTH receptor *(MCR2)* have been described in approximately 25% of these patients, most of which affect the trafficking of receptor molecules from the endoplasmic reticulum to the cell surface.
- Another 20% of cases are caused by mutations in *MRAP,* which encodes a melanocyte receptor accessory protein required for this trafficking.
- Mutations at new genetic loci have been identified, including the minichromosome maintenance-deficient four homolog *(MCM4)* and nicotinamide nucleotide transhydrogenase *(NNT).* These genes are involved in DNA replication and antioxidant defence, respectively.
- Patients with *MCM4* mutations also have growth failure, increased chromosomal breakage, and natural killer cell deficiency.
- Another syndrome of ACTH resistance occurs in association with achalasia of the gastric cardia and alacrima (triple A or Allgrove syndrome).
- These patients often have a progressive neurologic disorder that includes autonomic dysfunction, intellectual disability, motor neuropathy, and occasional deafness.
- This syndrome is also inherited in an autosomal recessive fashion, and the *AAAS* gene has

been mapped to chromosome 12q13. The encoded Aladin protein might help regulate nucleocytoplasmic transport of other proteins.

Type I Autoimmune Polyendocrinopathy Syndrome

- Although autoimmune Addison's disease most often occurs sporadically, it can occur as a component of 2 syndromes, each consisting of a constellation of autoimmune disorders.

- **Type I autoimmune polyendocrinopathy syndrome (APS-1),**

Also known as autoimmune polyendocrinopathy–candidiasis–ectodermal dystrophy (APECED) syndrome, it is inherited in a Mendelian autosomal recessive manner, whereas APS-2 has a complex inheritance pattern.

- **Chronic mucocutaneous candidiasis** is most often the first manifestation of APS-1, followed by hypoparathyroidism and then by Addison's disease, which typically develops in early adolescence.

- Other closely associated autoimmune disorders include gonadal failure, alopecia, vitiligo, keratopathy, enamel hypoplasia, nail dystrophy, intestinal malabsorption, and chronic active hepatitis. Hypothyroidism and type 1 diabetes mellitus occur in less than 10% of affected patients.
- Some components of the syndrome continue to develop as late as the fifth decade. Patients with APS-1 may have autoantibodies to the adrenal cytochrome P450 enzymes CYP21, CYP17, and CYP11A1.
- The presence of such antibodies indicates a high likelihood of the development of Addison's disease or, in female patients, ovarian failure.
- Adrenal failure can evolve rapidly in APS-1; death in patients with a previous diagnosis and unexplained deaths in siblings of patients with APS-1 have been reported, indicating the need to closely monitor patients with APS-1 (or any child with hypoparathyroidism of unknown aetiology) and to evaluate unaffected siblings of patients with this disorder thoroughly.

Disorders of Cholesterol Synthesis and Metabolism

- Patients with disorders of cholesterol synthesis or metabolism, including abetalipoproteinemia with deficient lipoprotein B-containing lipoproteins (such as low-density lipoprotein), and homozygous familial hypercholesterolemia, with impaired or absent low-density lipoprotein receptors, have mildly impaired adrenocortical function.
- Heterozygous familial hypercholesterolemia patients have normal adrenocortical function, unaffected by statin (HMG-CoA reductase inhibitor) treatment.
- Adrenal insufficiency has been reported in patients with Smith-Lemli-Opitz syndrome, an autosomal recessive disorder manifesting with facial anomalies, microcephaly, limb anomalies, and developmental delay. Mutations in the gene coding for sterol Δ7-Δ7-reductase, mapped to 11q12-q13, have been identified in Smith-Lemli-Opitz syndrome, resulting in impairment of the final step in cholesterol synthesis, with a marked elevation of 7-dehydrocholesterol, abnormally low cholesterol levels, and adrenal insufficiency.

- **Wolman disease**

It is a rare autosomal recessive disorder caused by mutations in the gene encoding human lysosomal acid lipase on chromosome 10q23.2 23.3. Cholesteryl esters accumulate in lysosomes in most organ systems, leading to organ failure. Infants during the first or second month of life have hepatosplenomegaly, steatorrhea, abdominal distention, and failure to thrive. Adrenal insufficiency and bilateral adrenal calcification are present, and death usually occurs in the 1st year of life.

Corticosteroid-Binding Globulin Deficiency and Decreased Cortisol-Binding Affinity

- Corticosteroid-binding globulin deficiency and decreased cortisol-binding affinity result in low plasma cortisol levels but normal urinary free cortisol and plasma ACTH levels.
- A high prevalence of hypotension and fatigue has been reported in some adults with corticosteroid-binding globulin deficiency.

Acquired Etiologies

- **Autoimmune Addison's Disease**

- The most common cause of Addison's disease is autoimmune destruction of the glands.

- The glands may be so small that they are not visible at autopsy, and only remnants of tissue are found in microscopic sections.
- Usually, the medulla is not destroyed, and there is marked lymphocytic infiltration in the area of the former cortex.
- In advanced disease, all adrenocortical function is lost, but isolated cortisol deficiency can occur early in the clinical course.
- Most patients have antiadrenal cytoplasmic antibodies in their plasma; 21-hydroxylase (CYP21) is the most commonly occurring biochemically defined autoantigen.
- Addison's disease can occur as a component of 2 autoimmune polyendocrinopathy syndromes.

- **Type II autoimmune polyendocrinopathy (APS-2)**

- It consists of Addison's disease associated with autoimmune thyroid disease (Schmidt syndrome) or type 1 diabetes (Carpenter syndrome).
- Gonadal failure, vitiligo, alopecia, and chronic atrophic gastritis, with or without pernicious anaemia, can occur.

- Frequencies of the human leukocyte antigen (HLA)-D3 and HLA-D4 alleles are increased in these patients and appear to confer an increased risk for development of this disease; particular alleles at the primary histocompatibility complex class I chain–related genes A and B *(MICA* and *MICB)* also are associated with this disorder.
- Polymorphisms in genes involved in other autoimmune disorders have been inconsistently associated with primary adrenal insufficiency, and their contribution to its pathogenesis must be regarded as uncertain.
- These include the class II, major histocompatibility complex, transactivator *(CIITA),* C-type lectin domain family 16, member A (*CLEC16A*), and protein tyrosine phosphatase, nonreceptor type 22 *(PTPN22).*
- The disorder is most common in middle-aged women and can occur in many generations of the same family. Anti-adrenal antibodies are also found in these patients, specifically antibodies to the CYP21, CYP17, and CYP11A1 enzymes. Autoimmune adrenal insufficiency may also be seen in patients with celiac disease and mitochondrial gene mutations.

- **Infection**
- Tuberculosis was a common cause of adrenal destruction in the past, but is currently much less prevalent. The most common infectious aetiology for adrenal insufficiency is meningococcemia; adrenal crisis from this cause is referred to as the Waterhouse-Friderichsen syndrome.
- Patients with AIDS can have a variety of subclinical abnormalities in the hypothalamic-pituitary-adrenal (HPA) axis, but frank adrenal insufficiency is rare. However, drugs used in the treatment of AIDS can affect adrenal hormone homeostasis.

Drugs

Ketoconazole,

An antifungal drug can cause adrenal insufficiency by inhibiting adrenal enzymes. Mitotane (o,p′-DDD), used in treating adrenocortical carcinoma and refractory Cushing syndrome, is cytotoxic to the adrenal cortex and can alter extra-adrenal cortisol metabolism. Signs of adrenal insufficiency occur in a substantial percentage of patients treated with mitotane.

- **Etomidate**,

Used in the induction and maintenance of general anaesthesia, inhibits 11β-hydroxylase (CYP11B1), and a single induction dose can block cortisol synthesis for 4-8 hr or longer. This may be problematic in severely stressed patients, particularly if repeated doses are used in a critical care setting.

- Abiraterone acetate, an androgen biosynthesis inhibitor which is used to treat metastatic prostate carcinoma, inhibits cortisol biosynthesis but leaves corticosterone biosynthesis unimpaired. This drug is not currently encountered in pediatric practice. Although not themselves a cause of adrenal insufficiency, rifampicin and anticonvulsive drugs such as phenytoin and phenobarbital reduce the effectiveness and bioavailability of corticosteroid replacement therapy by inducing steroid-metabolising enzymes in the liver.

- **Haemorrhage into Adrenal Glands**

Haemorrhage into the adrenal glands can occur in the neonatal period due to a difficult labour (especially breech presentation), or its aetiology might not be apparent. An incidence rate of 3 in 100,000 live births has been suggested.

- The haemorrhage may be sufficiently extensive to result in death from exsanguination or hypoadrenalism. An abdominal mass, anaemia, unexplained jaundice, or scrotal hematoma may be the presenting sign. Often, the haemorrhage is asymptomatic initially and is identified later by calcification of the adrenal gland. Foetal adrenal haemorrhage has also been reported.

- Postnatally, adrenal haemorrhage most often occurs in patients being treated with anticoagulants. It can also occur as a result of child abuse.

Clinical Manifestations

- Primary adrenal insufficiency leads to cortisol and often aldosterone deficiency.
- Cortisol deficiency decreases cardiac output and vascular tone; moreover, catecholamines such as epinephrine have decreased inotropic and pressor effects in the absence of cortisol.
- These problems are initially manifested as orthostatic hypotension in older children and can progress to frank shock in patients of any age.
- They are exacerbated by aldosterone deficiency, which results in hypovolemia owing to decreased resorption of sodium in the distal nephron.
- Hypotension and decreased cardiac output decrease glomerular filtration and thus the kidney's ability to excrete free water.
- The posterior pituitary secretes vasopressin (AVP) in response to hypotension and

also as a direct consequence of the lack of inhibition by cortisol.

- These factors decrease plasma osmolality and lead, in particular, to hyponatremia. Hyponatremia is also caused by aldosterone deficiency and may be much worse when both cortisol and aldosterone are deficient.
- In addition to hypovolemia and hyponatremia, aldosterone deficiency causes hyperkalemia by decreasing potassium excretion in the distal nephron. Cortisol deficiency alone does not cause hyperkalemia.
- Cortisol deficiency decreases negative feedback on the hypothalamus and pituitary, leading to increased secretion of ACTH.
- Hyperpigmentation is caused by ACTH and other peptide hormones (γ–melanocyte–stimulating hormone) arising from the ACTH precursor proopiomelanocortin. The skin can have a bronze cast in patients with a fair complexion. Pigmentation may be more prominent in skin creases, mucosa, and scars. In dark-skinned patients, it may be most readily appreciated in the gingival and buccal mucosa.
- Hypoglycemia is a feature of adrenal insufficiency. It is often accompanied by ketosis as the

body attempts to use fatty acids as an alternative energy source.

- Ketosis is aggravated by anorexia, nausea, and vomiting, all of which occur frequently. The clinical presentation of adrenal insufficiency depends on the patient's age, whether both cortisol and aldosterone secretion are affected, and, to some extent, on the underlying aetiology.
- Infants have a relatively greater requirement for aldosterone than older children, possibly owing to the kidneys' immaturity and the low sodium content of human breast milk and infant formula.
- Hyperkalemia, hyponatremia, and hypoglycemia are prominent presenting signs of adrenal insufficiency in infants.
- Ketosis is not consistently present because infants generate ketones less well than do older children.
- Hyperpigmentation is not usually seen because this takes weeks or months to develop, and orthostatic hypotension is challenging to demonstrate in infants.
- Infants can become ill very quickly. There may be only a few days of decreased activity,

anorexia, and vomiting before critical electrolyte abnormalities develop.

- In older children with Addison's disease, symptoms include muscle weakness, malaise, anorexia, vomiting, weight loss, and orthostatic hypotension.
- These may be of insidious onset.
- Such patients can present with acute decompensation (adrenal crisis) during relatively minor infectious illnesses.
- *Some of these patients have been initially misdiagnosed with chronic fatigue syndrome, postmononucleosis syndrome, chronic Lyme disease, or psychiatric disorders (depression or anorexia nervosa).*
- **Hyperpigmentation;**

is often, but not necessarily, present.

- **Hyponatremia**

It is present at diagnosis in almost 90% of patients.

- **Hyperkalaemia**

tends to occur later in the course of the disease in older children than in infants and is present in only half of the patients at diagnosis.

- *Normal potassium levels must never be presumed to rule out primary adrenal insufficiency.*
- Hypoglycemia and ketosis are common.

- The clinical presentation can be easily confused with gastroenteritis or other acute infections.
- Chronicity of symptoms can alert the clinician to the possibility of Addison's disease, but this diagnosis should be considered in any child with orthostatic hypotension, hyponatremia, hypoglycemia, and ketosis.
- Salt craving is seen in primary adrenal insufficiency with mineralocorticoid deficiency.
- Fatigue, myalgias, fever, eosinophilia, lymphocytosis, hypercalcemia, and anaemia may be noted with glucocorticoid deficiency.

Laboratory Findings

- An electrocardiogram is helpful for quickly detecting hyperkalemia in a critically ill child.
- Acidosis is often present, and the blood urea nitrogen level is elevated if the patient is dehydrated.
- Cortisol levels are sometimes at the low end of the normal range, but are invariably low when the patient's degree of illness is considered.
- ACTH levels are high in primary adrenal insufficiency, but can take time to be reported by the laboratory.

- Similarly, aldosterone levels may be within the normal range but inappropriately low considering the patient's hyponatremia, hyperkalemia, and hypovolemia. Plasma renin activity is elevated.
- The most definitive test for adrenal insufficiency is measurement of serum levels of cortisol before and after administration of ACTH; resting levels are low and do not typically increase after administration of ACTH. Occasionally, normal resting levels that do not improve after administration of
- ACTH indicate an absence of adrenocortical reserve. A low initial level followed by a significant response to ACTH can indicate secondary adrenal insufficiency.
- Traditionally, this test measured cortisol levels before and 30 or 60 minutes after giving 0.250 mg of cosyntropin (ACTH 1-24) by rapid intravenous infusion.
- Aldosterone will transiently increase in response to this dose of ACTH and may also be measured. A low-dose test (1 µg ACTH 1- 24/1.73 m2) is a more sensitive test of pituitary-adrenal reserve but has somewhat lower specificity (more false-positive tests). Ultrasonography (which requires

an experienced operator), CT, or MRI can help to define the size of the adrenal glands.

Differential Diagnosis

- Upon presentation, Addison's disease often needs to be distinguished from more acute illnesses such as gastroenteritis with dehydration or sepsis.
- Additional testing is directed at identifying the specific cause of adrenal insufficiency.
- When congenital adrenal hyperplasia is suspected, serum levels of cortisol precursors (17-hydroxyprogesterone) should be measured along with cortisol in an ACTH stimulation test.
- Elevated levels of very-long-chain fatty acids are diagnostic of ALD.
- Many genetic etiologies for primary adrenal insufficiency may be identified by direct genetic testing, but results can take many weeks to become available. The presence of antiadrenal antibodies suggests an autoimmune pathogenesis.
- Patients with autoimmune Addison's disease must be closely observed for the development of other autoimmune disorders.
- In children, hypoparathyroidism is the most commonly associated disorder, and it is

suspected if hypocalcemia and elevated phosphate levels are present.

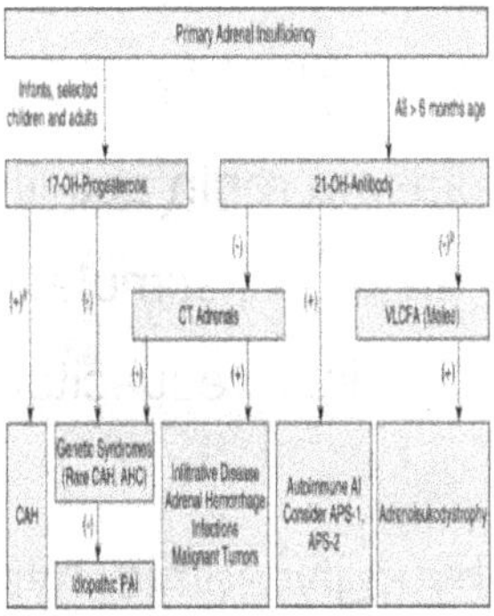

Treatment

Treatment of acute adrenal insufficiency must be *immediate and vigorous.* If the diagnosis of adrenal insufficiency has not been established, a blood sample should be obtained before therapy to determine electrolytes, glucose, ACTH, cortisol, aldosterone, and plasma renin activity. If the patient's condition permits, an ACTH stimulation test can be performed while initial fluid resuscitation is underway.

To correct hypoglycaemia, hypovolemia, and hyponatremia, an intravenous solution of 5% glucose in 0.9% saline should be administered.

Hypotonic fluids (e.g., 5% glucose in water or 0.2% saline) must be avoided because they can precipitate or exacerbate hyponatremia.

If hyperkalaemia is severe, it can require treatment with intravenous calcium and/or bicarbonate, intrarectal potassium-binding resin (sodium polystyrene sulfonate, Kayexalate), or intravenous infusion of glucose and insulin.

- A water-soluble form of hydrocortisone, such as hydrocortisone sodium succinate, should be given intravenously. For infants, 10 mg; for toddlers, 25 mg; for older children, 50 mg; and for adolescents, 100 mg should be administered as a bolus. A similar total amount should be given in divided doses at 6-hour intervals for the first 24 hours.
- These doses may be reduced during the next 24 hr if progress is satisfactory.
- Adequate fluid and sodium repletion is achieved by intravenous saline administration, aided by the mineralocorticoid effect of high doses of hydrocortisone.

Particular caution should be exercised in the rare patient with concomitant adrenal insufficiency and hypothyroidism, because thyroxine can increase cortisol clearance, and an adrenal crisis may be precipitated if hypothyroidism is treated without first ensuring adequate glucocorticoid replacement.

After the acute manifestations are under control, most patients require chronic replacement therapy for their cortisol and aldosterone deficiencies.

Hydrocortisone (cortisol) may be administered orally in daily doses of 10 $mg/m^2/24$ hr in three divided doses; some patients require 15 $mg/m^2/24$ hr to minimise fatigue, especially in the morning.

Equivalent doses (20–25% of the hydrocortisone dose) of prednisone or prednisolone may be divided and given twice daily. ACTH levels may be used to monitor adequacy of glucocorticoid replacement in primary adrenal insufficiency; in congenital adrenal hyperplasia, levels of precursor hormones are used instead. Blood samples for monitoring should be obtained at a consistent time of day and in a consistent relation to (i.e., before or after) the hydrocortisone dose.

Morning ACTH levels in the normal range, 3-4 times normal, are satisfactory.

Untreated or severely undertreated patients can acutely decompensate during relatively minor illnesses; assessment of symptoms (or lack thereof) must not be used as a substitute for biochemical monitoring.

During situations of stress, such as periods of infection or minor surgical procedures, the dose of hydrocortisone should be increased 2-3 3 times. Major surgery under general inhalation anaesthesia requires high intravenous doses of hydrocortisone similar to those used for acute adrenal insufficiency.

If aldosterone deficiency is present, fludrocortisone, a synthetic mineralocorticoid, is given orally in doses of 0.05-0.2 mg daily.

Measurements of plasma renin activity help monitor the adequacy of mineralocorticoid replacement. Chronic overdosage with glucocorticoids leads to obesity, short stature, and osteoporosis, whereas overdosage with fludrocortisone results in hypertension and occasionally hypokalaemia.

Chapter 6

Trauma and Emergency Nursing

questions

Content

1. Severe facial injuries, for example, those resulting from going through a windshield, increase the risk for all of the following. For which complication would you assess first?

2. Which drug treatment helps to decrease ICP by expanding plasma and the osmotic effect of moving fluid?

How It Works:

Signs and symptoms

Observing

- Application of RICE (rest, ice, compression, and elevation) is indicated for initial management of which type of injury?

Breakdown of RICE for Injury Management

Examples of Injuries Where RICE is Applied

Limitations of RICE

- You are performing abdominal thrusts on a 9-year-old child when he suddenly becomes unresponsive. After you shout for help from nearby, what is the most appropriate action to take?

Call for Emergency Help

Lay the Child on a Flat Surface

Check for Breathing and Pulse

Initiate Chest Compressions

Give Rescue Breaths

Check for Foreign Objects in the Mouth

Severe facial injuries, for example, those resulting from going through a windshield, increase the risk for all of the following. For which complication would you assess first?

The most critical and pressing issues to take into account while evaluating a patient who has sustained significant facial injuries from trauma, such as being struck by a car, are as follows:

- Blockage of the airways
- Bleeding
- Damage to the cervical spine
- Instance of infection
- Loss or impairment of vision

Out of all these, airway obstruction is the problem that needs to be evaluated initially. Trauma to the face can cause aspiration of vomit, swelling, bleeding, and displacement of facial tissues, all of which can obstruct the airway. It becomes a potentially fatal condition. Mandibular or midface fractures from facial trauma may force tissues backwards into the neck, blocking airflow. Blood from cuts or fractured facial bones can also build up in the airway, making breathing difficult or even fatal.

The following actions are taken to evaluate airway obstruction:

- Visual examination of the lips and face immediately for signs of swelling, blood, or foreign objects.
- Listen for unusual breathing noises, such as stridor, gurgling, or wheezing, which could be signs of partial obstruction.
- Monitor the patient's level of consciousness, skin tone, and oxygen saturation, as hypoxia can strike suddenly.
- If a cervical spine injury is suspected, opening the airway without moving the neck can be accomplished by performing a jaw thrust or chin raise.

Other issues, such as bleeding, cervical spine injuries, and visual impairment, should be addressed after making sure the airway is secure.

Which drug treatment helps to decrease ICP by expanding plasma and the osmotic effect of moving fluid?

Mannitol, an osmotic diuretic, is a medication that expands plasma and uses an osmotic effect to transfer fluid to help

lower intracranial pressure (ICP), reduce brain oedema and lower ICP. Mannitol works by removing water from the brain tissues and putting it into circulation.

How It Works:

- Mannitol produces an osmotic gradient since it does not penetrate the blood-brain barrier.
- Reduced brain oedema results from this gradient's fluid drawing into the vascular space from the brain's intracellular and extracellular spaces.
- Plasma expansion improves cerebral blood flow, which may lessen ischemia arising when ICP is raised.

Signs and symptoms

- Patients with brain tumours, traumatic brain injury, stroke, and other disorders where elevated ICP is a concern are frequently treated with mannitol.

- It is usually used in acute situations where a quick drop in ICP is necessary.

Observing

- Since mannitol therapy might result in hyperosmolarity and electrolyte imbalances, it is imperative to monitor serum osmolality and electrolytes.
- It is crucial to monitor urine production because mannitol has a diuretic effect that can cause dehydration if lost fluid is not sufficiently restored.

Due to its osmotic properties, mannitol remains one of the most widely used and effective treatments for reducing intracranial pressure (ICP), while hypertonic saline is another option.

Application of RICE (rest, ice, compression, and elevation) is indicated for initial management of which type of injury?

The RICE method, which stands for rest, ice, compression, and elevation, is primarily indicated for the initial management of acute musculoskeletal injuries, such as:

- Sprains: Ligament injuries caused by the stretching or tearing of ligaments, commonly seen in the ankle, wrist, or knee.
- Strains are Muscle or tendon injuries that often occur in the lower back or the hamstrings.
- Contusions: Bruises caused by direct trauma to muscles or soft tissues.
- Minor fractures (until further medical evaluation)

Breakdown of RICE for Injury Management

1. Rest: Immobilising the injured area prevents further damage to the affected ligaments, tendons, or muscles and begins the healing process.
2. Ice: Applying cold to the injured area reduces swelling and pain by constricting blood vessels and limiting the inflammatory response. Ice

should be applied for 20-30 minutes every 2-3 hours during the first 48 hours after the injury.

3. Compression: Wrapping the injured area with an elastic bandage or compression wrap helps limit swelling and supports the injured structure. The compression should be snug but not so tight that it restricts blood flow.

4. Elevation: Keeping the injured limb above heart level minimises swelling by promoting venous return of blood from the wounded site, reducing fluid accumulation.

Examples of Injuries Where RICE is Applied

- Ankle sprain: A common injury where the ligaments of the ankle are overstretched, leading to pain, swelling, and limited mobility.
- A hamstring strain occurs when the muscles at the back of the thigh are overstretched or torn, often from running or quick movements.
- Knee sprain or strain: Injuries to the ligaments or tendons of the knee, often resulting from sudden twisting motions.

Limitations of RICE

- RICE effectively manages soft tissue injuries during the acute phase (the first 48-72 hours).

Still, it is not a definitive treatment for more severe injuries, such as complete ligament tears or fractures. Further medical evaluation, imaging, and possibly surgical intervention may be required.

- **You are performing abdominal thrusts on a 9-year-old child when he suddenly becomes unresponsive. After you shout for help from nearby, what is the most appropriate action to take?**

When a 9-year-old child becomes unresponsive while you are performing abdominal thrusts due to choking, it is crucial to act immediately. The following steps should be taken:

Call for Emergency Help

- Immediately shout for nearby help and ensure that emergency medical services (EMS) are being called. Instruct someone specifically to call 911 or the appropriate emergency number if others are around.

7. **Lay the Child on a Flat Surface**

- Place the child on their back on a firm, flat surface, such as the floor.

8. **Check for Breathing and Pulse**

- Quickly assess whether the child is breathing or has any signs of life (e.g., moving or coughing).

- Check the child's pulse (usually at the carotid artery in the neck for a child this age) for no more than 10 seconds.

9. **Initiate Chest Compressions**

If there is no breathing or pulse, or the pulse is less than 60 beats per minute, and there are signs of poor perfusion (e.g., pale, cold skin), begin cardiopulmonary resuscitation (CPR) immediately. It is done as follows:

- Start with chest compressions: Use the heel of one hand to perform compressions in the centre of the child's chest, between the nipples.
- Push hard and fast: Compress the chest at least one-third of the depth of about 2 inches (5 cm) at a rate of 100-120 compressions per minute. Allow the chest to recoil completely between compressions.

10. **Give Rescue Breaths**

- After 30 compressions, give two rescue breaths.
- Tilt the child's head slightly and lift the chin to open the airway.
- Pinch the child's nose, make a seal over the child's mouth with yours, and deliver a breath just enough to make the chest rise.
- If the chest does not rise, reposition the head and try again.

11. **Check for Foreign Objects in the Mouth**

- After each set of compressions and before taking a breath, open the child's mouth to see if the object causing the obstruction is visible.
- If you see the object, carefully attempt to remove it with a finger sweep, not pushing it further back into the airway.
- If you cannot see the object, do not perform a blind finger sweep, which can cause further blockage.

Chapter 7

Trauma

Content

Priority Decision:

During the primary survey, the nurse identified asymmetric chest wall movement in the patient. What intervention should the nurse first perform?

Immediate First Intervention:

Administer Supplemental Oxygen

Additional Steps Based on Findings

Call for Emergency Assistance

Prepare for Intubation or Mechanical Ventilation (If Necessary)

Perform Needle Decompression for Suspected Tension Pneumothorax

Assist with Chest Tube Insertion

Immobilise Flail Chest (If Applicable)

Continuous Monitoring

Rationale

Why must the nurse obtain details of the incident during the secondary survey of a trauma patient in the Emergency Department?

b) Guiding Focused Assessment and Treatment

Identifying Hidden or Delayed Injuries

c) Informing Multidisciplinary Teams and Specialist Consultations

Establishing the Context of Trauma for Preventive Measures

e) Assessing the Severity and Predicting Patient Outcomes

Providing Legal and Forensic Evidence

g) Ensuring Emotional and Psychological Support

During the primary survey, the nurse identified asymmetric chest wall movement in the patient. What intervention should the nurse first perform?

Asymmetric chest wall movement during the primary survey indicates a potential serious injury, such as a flail chest, or underlying conditions, like a pneumothorax, both of which can impair breathing and lead to respiratory failure. The nurse's first intervention should stabilise the patient's respiratory function.

Immediate First Intervention:

Administer Supplemental Oxygen

The first step is to ensure adequate oxygenation. The nurse should immediately administer high-flow oxygen using a non-rebreather mask or another appropriate delivery method to improve oxygen saturation. It helps maintain tissue oxygenation while further assessment and interventions are conducted.

Additional Steps Based on Findings

Once oxygen is provided, further interventions may include:

Call for Emergency Assistance

The nurse should immediately alert the trauma or emergency medical team. Asymmetric chest wall movement suggests a potentially life-threatening condition, and immediate medical attention is crucial.

Prepare for Intubation or Mechanical Ventilation (If Necessary)

If the patient's oxygenation does not improve or respiratory distress worsens, intubation and mechanical ventilation may be necessary to maintain oxygenation. It is imperative in the event of a significant respiratory compromise.

Perform Needle Decompression for Suspected Tension Pneumothorax

Suppose the patient shows signs of tension pneumothorax (e.g., absent breath sounds on one side, tracheal deviation, hypotension). In that case, the nurse should prepare for an immediate needle decompression, which a physician or an advanced practice nurse typically performs. Needle decompression involves inserting a large-bore needle into the second intercostal space at the midclavicular line to relieve the pressure.

Assist with Chest Tube Insertion

If a pneumothorax or hemothorax is confirmed, the nurse should assist the healthcare provider with inserting a chest tube. This intervention will help re-expand the lung and resolve the underlying cause of the asymmetric chest movement.

Immobilise Flail Chest (If Applicable)

If a flail chest is suspected (where two or more consecutive ribs are fractured in multiple places), the nurse may need to stabilise the chest wall with the use of supportive dressings or splints.

Mechanical ventilation, also known as positive pressure ventilation, may be required in severe cases.

Continuous Monitoring

The nurse should closely monitor the patient's respiratory rate, effort, and oxygen saturation. Any deterioration in the condition must be communicated promptly to the medical team.

Monitoring vital signs, particularly oxygen saturation and heart rate, will help assess the effectiveness of interventions.

Rationale

Asymmetric chest wall movement is a critical finding because it often indicates impaired ventilation, which can lead to hypoxia and respiratory failure. Administering high-flow oxygen ensures that the patient's tissues are adequately oxygenated while more definitive treatment is being arranged. Following this, the nurse's role includes monitoring and assisting with interventions like chest tube insertion or intubation to resolve the underlying cause. Ensuring proper oxygenation and respiratory support is always the top priority in cases involving compromised breathing mechanics. By addressing the respiratory distress first, the nurse can prevent further deterioration of the patient's condition while ensuring that advanced interventions are prepared for or performed as soon as possible.

Why must the nurse obtain details of the incident during the secondary survey of a trauma patient in the Emergency Department?

The secondary survey in trauma care is a systematic and comprehensive assessment performed after the patient has been stabilised following the primary survey (which focuses on life-threatening conditions such as airway, breathing, circulation, and neurological deficits). During the secondary survey, the nurse collects detailed information about the trauma, focusing on understanding the extent of the injuries and any underlying or complicating factors that could affect the patient's care. Obtaining incident details during this stage is crucial for several reasons, outlined below:

c) Guiding Focused Assessment and Treatment

Understanding the mechanism of injury (MOI) and how the trauma occurred allows healthcare professionals to anticipate specific injuries. For example, if the trauma resulted from a high-velocity car accident, the nurse would look for injuries consistent with blunt trauma, such as internal bleeding, fractures, or spinal cord damage. Alternatively, a penetrating trauma from a gunshot or stabbing may lead to a different injury pattern, such as damage to specific organs, vascular structures, or bones. By knowing the MOI, the nurse can tailor the assessment to potential injuries that might not be immediately obvious but are likely given the incident's nature. This knowledge helps prioritise diagnostics such as imaging or laboratory tests and ensures timely and appropriate treatment.

b) Identifying Hidden or Delayed Injuries

Many injuries may not be apparent during the primary survey and may not become evident until later. Some injuries, like intracranial bleeding, splenic rupture, or internal organ damage, may manifest later. By gathering detailed information about the incident, the nurse can keep a higher index of suspicion for such injuries. For example, in a fall from a height, the nurse should assess for long bone fractures, spinal cord injuries, or internal organ damage, even if the patient appears stable initially. Similarly, knowing the speed and impact of a car crash can indicate the likelihood of internal injuries, even in the absence of external wounds. This information enables the nurse to initiate serial monitoring or conduct further diagnostic tests, such as computed tomography (CT) scans or X-rays, to detect evolving conditions.

c) Informing Multidisciplinary Teams and Specialist Consultations

Details about the trauma incident are critical for effective communication among the trauma team, including physicians, surgeons, and specialists (e.g., orthopaedic or neurosurgeons). By relaying information about the MOI and other details, the nurse ensures that all team members are informed and can participate in developing the patient's care plan. For instance, in a multi-system trauma patient, the details of a crush injury from a building collapse might prompt the early involvement of orthopaedic surgeons, general surgeons, and even plastic surgeons if there is extensive soft tissue damage. Likewise, knowledge of a blast injury from an explosion may necessitate consultations with specialists in burns or respiratory care, as the patient might have sustained inhalation injuries.

d) Establishing the Context of Trauma for Preventive Measures

Understanding how the trauma occurred can also provide context for counselling and prevention strategies. For instance, if the trauma resulted from a workplace accident, such as a fall due to a lack of safety equipment, the nurse can notify occupational safety authorities to prevent future incidents. In cases of domestic violence or child abuse, the details of the incident may raise red flags, allowing the nurse to involve social workers, legal authorities, or protective services for the patient's safety.

e) Assessing the Severity and Predicting Patient Outcomes

Incident details can provide insight into the severity of the trauma, which helps predict the likely course of treatment and recovery. For example, a patient involved in a high-impact motor vehicle collision (MVC) is more likely to have severe injuries, longer recovery times, and a higher risk of complications than someone involved in a low-impact incident. The details of the trauma inform the healthcare team of the expected injury severity and prognosis, aiding in counselling the patient and family about the potential treatment trajectory and outcomes.

f) Providing Legal and Forensic Evidence

In some cases, such as assaults, vehicular accidents, or industrial injuries, the trauma incident becomes part of a legal or forensic investigation.

Gathering accurate and comprehensive details about the trauma can be essential for law enforcement or legal proceedings. The nurse's documentation of the injury, including the patient's account of the event and observations, can serve as evidence in court cases or workplace injury claims. In these cases, the nurse's role extends to accurately recording the circumstances of the injury, preserving proof (such as clothing or foreign objects), and maintaining a transparent chain of custody for forensic materials.

g) Ensuring Emotional and Psychological Support

Trauma is not only a physical experience but also an emotional and psychological one. By obtaining detailed information about the incident, the nurse gains insight into the patient's emotional state and potential need for mental health support. For instance, if the trauma was related to violence or a traumatic accident, the nurse may need to involve mental health services, such as counselling or psychiatric evaluation, to help the patient cope with emotional trauma and post-traumatic stress disorder (PTSD). The nurse's understanding of the incident provides the foundation for compassionate and holistic care that addresses physical and emotional needs.

In summary, obtaining incident details during the secondary survey of a trauma patient is critical to guiding a comprehensive assessment, identifying hidden injuries, facilitating communication with the trauma team, informing legal investigations, and providing psychological support. It ensures that the nurse and healthcare team deliver patient-centred, informed, and timely care, optimising the patient's short- and long-term outcomes.

Chapter 8

Veterans Access to Care Department of Veterans Affairs Health Care.

Content

Veterans Access to Care Department of Veterans Affairs Health Care

Veterans are among the most important servants of American society, having fought for the United States to restore the ideologies and principles that the people of the American community enjoy today. The Department of Veterans Affairs (VA) Healthcare is also a vital healthcare system that has been established to provide the services that are required by veterans, especially for those who survive the devastating effects of wars within and outside the United States in military missions. The Armed Forces of the United States stand at the top of the notch in defending the country's territory and ensuring the citizens ' safety in terms of their lives and their social and economic welfare. However, Veterans have been found to encounter numerous challenges in their attempts to access healthcare services from the VA. The research report examines the challenges that veterans face in accessing quality and efficient healthcare services from the VA, particularly among rural veterans. It identifies areas that require improvement and outlines new initiatives that must be implemented to provide comprehensive, high-quality care to U.S. veterans.

Problem Formulation

Various issues have hindered access to healthcare services from the VA. These issues range from the lack of accessibility to the healthcare facilities that provide healthcare to veteran patients, the strict eligibility criteria that lead to discrimination against some service men and women, the disparities in care delivery, and inadequate mental health services. (Van Slyke & Armstrong, 2020). The most significant concern for American veterans has been the issue of cognitive issues that not only hinder access to required quality services but also constrain the diversification of services to meet the needs of individual veterans. Lack of personnel and challenges with technology are additional factors that have been identified as hindering soldiers' access to VA healthcare services. (Jones et al., 2020)Like other servants, soldiers have families that depend on them for provision. These veterans may be constrained by budgetary issues related to accessing their healthcare services. Fiscal constraints may limit accessibility to medical services, as other structural barriers and inequalities result from aspects such as ethnicity and cultural diversity, which are closely correlated with the economic welfare of veteran members. (Ofori, 2020)One critical issue that has been found to affect veterans is the dispersion of VA facilities, in the sense that sometimes they are not accessible to the veterans when they are needed. This contributes to budgetary constraints, as the far-off soldiers may not readily and quickly access the VA, as the accessibility costs are not covered. The veterans, therefore, end up in desperate situations where they cannot access veteran services due to multiple challenges.

Access to non-VA care expansion was among the strategies that increased veterans' access to community hospitals, which are funded by Medicaid and the Department of Veterans Affairs (VA). The literature review identifies a significant reduction in the number of veterans who utilised the VA services and facilities. (Peterson et al., 2018)The critical shift from VA hospitals to community-based facilities did not affect mortality rates. The crucial challenge that requires evaluation and comprehension is why, despite the diversification of Medicaid to cover community-based hospitals, many veterans still opt to use VA hospitals.

The 2014 US VA MISSION Act aimed to increase access to community care, allowing accessibility challenges and structural, economic, and psychological barriers to be quickly addressed. However, this was another contributing factor to the trends observed in this study, as veterans continued to prefer VA healthcare over private community hospitals. (Peterson et al., 2018)Therefore, the critical concern remains whether increasing access to personal care would reduce veterans' challenges regarding access to healthcare. Coordinating inpatient care when veterans are transitioning from the VA to non-VA hospitals is challenging for clinicians and the general healthcare system. (Ayele et al., 2021). Stakeholders have been required to reevaluate the transition process to ensure that the key aim of enhancing quality and patient outcomes through increased accessibility is achieved. The systems also aim to diversify the issues that the veterans face, rather than generalising them, so that those who do not have economic and social advantages can access the same quality of services to improve their health outcomes. The fundamental strategy for the healthcare system is to have a clear statement of its objectives and the guidelines that would achieve these goals. Additionally, issues such as generating profits, educating healthcare professionals about the challenges facing veterans, enhancing administrative structures, and responding to political pressures may limit the constraints on healthcare service delivery to veterans. The ultimate goal is to restore the veterans' everyday social life and ensure they are happy with their families and satisfied with their health conditions.

Rationale and Motivations for the Study

One critical concern that may motivate this study is the growing concern about the quality of healthcare that Veterans receive from the VA. The number of veterans across the United States has been increasing, and the trend has been upward. (Hunt et al., 2019). Veterans have faced numerous challenges, especially in accessing government healthcare services, since they serve the people of the United States. With mental issues being among the most significant and most observable issues that require unique and quality medical attention, other problems that the VA could address go down to the welfare of the Veteran's social and economic welfare. For instance, the treatment of Post Traumatic Stress Disorder (PTSD), anxiety, depression, and drug and substance addiction can be crucial in restoring the economic and social life of veterans. (Mobbs &

Bonanno, 2018)The therapy and counselling sessions can help the veterans find employment, support their families, and restore their relationships with other members of society.

The veterans have encountered various challenges in accessing VA healthcare services, resulting in delayed and low-quality services for these vital social service providers. Veterans have been found to experience long wait times, restricted access to special services, which are essentially supposed to be diverse, and delays in the provision of treatment services. (Jones et al., 2020). These challenges have resulted in the worsening of healthcare conditions in cases where injuries are involved, anxiety about the uncertainty of health, and the death of soldiers. Individuals with complex medical conditions are among the veterans who are most affected, since some mental concerns and physical health issues require adequate and immediate medical attention. The accessibility of healthcare services within the VA motivates investigations to understand the systemic challenges that the VA experiences in delivering services to veterans. Mismanagement, inadequate staffing of healthcare physicians and specialists, and economic constraints due to insufficient resources are among the key underlying factors contributing to the inaccessibility of healthcare services. (Ayele et al., 2021)Understanding the VA system framework is challenging due to its complexity. It is the most complicated and integrated healthcare system in the United States. Understanding the network between inpatient and outpatient services comprises one of the holistic frameworks for addressing veterans' challenges in seeking quality and timely healthcare services.

Policy changes and system adjustments to make healthcare accessible to all veterans, from the diversity of their socio-cultural, economic, and personal perspectives, would ensure that they have timely and appropriate access to the healthcare they need. (Ofori, 2020). One of the critical issues is that healthcare providers face challenges in addressing the specific needs of veterans due to knowledge gaps in their care. Some of the challenges that require special care are service-related injuries of the soldiers and some wild combination of mental conditions that may make the soldiers unfit to co-exist with other members of the community. Sometimes, the soldiers struggle to transition from the battlefields to a typical lifestyle. For example, they require help settling down, finding suitable jobs, acquiring new skills, starting families, or reestablishing lost connections with their families. Essentially, the challenges are more specific and diverse, and soldiers cannot be satisfied with the services offered in community hospitals, as the challenges veterans face are different. Some veterans are homeless due to the inability to cope with the economic pressures and despair of living an everyday life. The motivation for conducting this study is to understand the issues of comprehensive eligibility criteria, geographical barriers, logistics, and social and economic factors that impact service delivery.

Research Questions/Hypotheses

R1. What are the challenges and barriers to VA healthcare access for rural Veterans?

R2. How do the challenges and barriers to VA healthcare access influence veterans' quality of healthcare and well-being?

R3. What are potential solutions to enhancing timely and comprehensive quality VA healthcare access for rural Veterans?

H10. There are no significant challenges or barriers to VA healthcare access for rural Veterans

H10. There are significant challenges and barriers to VA healthcare access for rural Veterans.

H20. How do the challenges and barriers to VA healthcare access influence veterans' quality of healthcare and well-being?

H2A. How do the challenges and barriers to VA healthcare access influence veterans' quality of healthcare and well-being?

H30. There are no potential solutions to enhancing timely and comprehensive access to VA healthcare for rural Veterans.

H3A. There are potential solutions to enhancing timely and comprehensive access to VA healthcare for rural Veterans.

Purpose and Objectives

The study aims to identify the barriers that have constrained veterans' access to healthcare within the VA system in remote and rural locations. Veterans in rural, remote settings have struggled for a long time to access diversified inpatient care from the VA system. The barriers have been exacerbated by distance, technical challenges within the VA facilities, and staffing issues. The research hypothesises that staffing and technological barriers are among the key challenges that hinder the VA system within rural settings from offering high-quality services. These factors increased appointment wait times, especially for patients needing critical medical services, and limited access to specialised care. This study aims to identify the barriers to accessing quality VA healthcare, understand how these challenges impact the quality of care, and develop strategies to enhance timely and comprehensive quality care for veteran patients in remote areas.

Concepts Related to the Study

Comprehending the concepts related to this study is a critical measure in completing the survey, as it constrains the research to a precise scope. The most significant idea is understanding the meaning of the Veterans' Healthcare Administration (VA Healthcare). This is a body that the United States established to provide healthcare services to veterans. Some of the services that VA Health Care offers are highly specialised care for injured veterans, mental care, rehabilitation from issues such as addiction to drugs, and therapy for soldiers to enhance transition from military life to a typical social and economic lifestyle.

Accessing VA Medical Care refers to the ease and convenience with which veterans can access available services. Some factors that may hinder accessibility include geographical location, transportation, logistics to reach VA Healthcare institutions, longer wait times, and eligibility requirements. Other underlying aspects include the cultural barriers that not only constrain active accessibility but also limit the availability of services in some remote areas. A critical analysis and examination of these barriers is essential for developing the desired quality and comprehensive VA healthcare system that addresses and overcomes these challenges.

Excellent care is another critical concept surrounding quality, efficiency, and efficacy. The concept used in this context refers to the degree of compliance of VA Healthcare services with established standards or expectations. Studies have cited the level of compliance and quality of VA Health services to raise contentious debates in society about the type of services that should be delivered to American veterans compared to non-VA services. The VA is substandard, yet the veterans have always prioritised it.

Veterans' demographic information refers to the characteristics that define the population composition of Veterans. These features include age, gender, ethnic affiliation, and disabilities. While demographic information describes the individual composition of veterans, it provides a starting point for comprehending why VA health services do not meet the needs of the particular demographic composition.

Mental Wellness: In the context of veterans, mental wellness refers to their mental health. The Veterans face numerous challenges while executing their duties as soldiers in the US military. As such, the veterans have encountered risky situations ranging from anxiety from the uncertainty of what may transpire to worse traumatic encounters leading to mental health disorders like PTSD, substance abuse, and depression. Mental wellness necessitates providing healthcare services depending on the severity of the conditions.

Health Results: The health result is a concept that contextualises how VA healthcare services help patients achieve treatment outcomes. The overall health results are expected to be observed by restoring normal physiological and mental functioning in the veterans' bodily systems, allowing them to lead an everyday life like non-veterans. The comprehension of the health results desired by veterans is vital in understanding the efficiency of health systems in meeting patients' needs.

The price of care refers to the shared cost required to achieve the standard quality of care for veterans and the VA healthcare system. A critical point to note from the outset of this research is that healthcare services are offered at a cost because they are not free. The price ranges from the resources that should be invested for that purpose, including developing facilities and infrastructure, hiring personnel such as specialists, and paying for the required equipment. The costs, therefore, are essentially the financial burden that the veterans and the VA should incur in offering the services.

The comparison to non-VA healthcare examines the quality of services offered by VA healthcare systems in relation to those provided by non-VA healthcare, considering the differing demographic compositions of former military personnel. Comparing the non-VA system to the VA system provides a clear overview of the strengths, weaknesses, and areas that require improvement to ensure that veterans have access to quality services.

Patient-centeredness refers to providing services that align with the immediate needs of veterans. For instance, military personnel undergo different experiences while serving the country. Since these experiences differ due to underlying factors such as cultural differences, economic status, and numerous other issues, the healthcare systems through the VA require comprehensive services tailored to the patient's level of need.

Limitations and Ethical Considerations

The research may be limited to a narrow scope and may not apply to other areas that were not investigated. Although the research aims to provide a comprehensive overview of the challenges veterans face in accessing VA healthcare services, the study may not address the views of veterans in other regions within the United States, as healthcare access policies differ from one state to another. The research methodology and design may limit the findings, as they may not involve collecting data from a broader range and depth, which could hinder the identification of barriers and potential solutions that may be required. The research may experience challenges drawing causal inferences, and the ambulatory data may be concealed or unavailable.

The available data may not be dependable because soldiers' experiences may be traumatic, and respondents may conceal some information. The data sources may present a general view of what has been discovered. It may not accurately represent the actual issues that veterans are facing, considering that they experience different challenges. The accessibility, availability, and reliability of data, therefore, may be a limitation to drawing accurate conclusions.

The ethical considerations for this study will involve upholding the highest form of integrity, whereby the research will focus on the transparent relaying of findings and methods in data collection. Since the lives of veterans are a sensitive issue, the approaches to collecting and analysing will uphold the participants' privacy. The names will not be disclosed in the results discussion. Conflicts of interest will be avoided to ensure that the research is not predetermined or biased based on the researcher's experiences. Collecting data and communicating the findings must restore respect to the veterans and the stakeholders involved in providing healthcare services through the VA healthcare system.

Literature Review

Reasons for Selection of Literature

The Veterans Health Administration (VHA) is an organisation within the United States committed to providing healthcare services to different demographic compositions of veterans, including individuals from various ethnic backgrounds, ages, and genders. The VA has made significant progress in enhancing the delivery and access to quality veteran-centric care by prioritising the views and diverse needs of the veterans in guiding the establishment of comprehensive healthcare. (Cheney et al., 2018). However, some veterans have faced multiple challenges in accessing VA healthcare services. There has been little attention paid to the prior military service of the veterans and the daily struggles of the veterans, especially when they seek mental health services. About one million soldiers who had been deployed to Iraq and Afghanistan had experienced challenges transitioning back to their everyday lives in the United States by 2018. The projection was that they would do so within the next five years (Mobbs & Bonanno, 2018). The transition was an issue because military engagement varied depending on the duration of service commitment and their age, making it difficult to track how many were affected in the risk groups. Mobbs and Bonanno (2018) found that transitioning from veterans who require mental health services was the result of sociocultural issues, such as stigmatisation from non-veteran civilians. Cheney et al. (2018) noted that the function of the VA was to enhance equitable access to healthcare by eliminating factors that may contribute to inequality, such as stigmatisation as a social issue. The Office of Health Equity is responsible for eliminating health disparities based on the diversity of the veterans. The Office of Health Equity-QUERI Partnered Evaluation Centre serves as an oversight body for evaluating healthcare quality provided through the VA system, with a focus on the most pressing issues, including gender, geographic location, and minority ethnic groups.

Overview of Rural Veterans

Rural veterans form a significant number of soldiers who have served in the military. Cheney et al. (2018) note that about 4.7 rural veterans, more than half of this number, use the VA health system. However, rural settings have experienced disparities in accessibility and quality of services. The rural veteran population has had more restricted access to VA healthcare than the urban and suburban groups. (Cyr et al., 2019). The majority of the rural dwellers are veterans with low education levels in rural settings where there are higher poverty rates. The rural population mainly comprises older individuals, who are less likely to experience long delays and incomplete accessibility to medical services, a common problem in the United States, especially in rural areas. Cheney et al. (2018), for instance, found that Hollis, Alaska, was the nearest VA healthcare system facility, which was more than 1,000 miles away. These raise concerns over how fast the veterans can access emergency services in critical conditions and the disadvantage of the rural population that is economically suppressed.

Mental Health

Mental health care access has been under scrutiny, particularly in terms of its affordability for patients in rural and underserved suburban areas. Meffert et al. (2019) found that the Affordable Care Act does not expand its coverage and benefits for low-income individuals. It is vital to consider the study by Cyr et al. (2019), which suggests that the rural population comprises more people who are poor with limited earnings. The new law contains a disadvantage to the rural populations in that mental healthcare cannot be covered under the comprehensive care plan. According to Meffert et al. (2019), there are systemic disparities whereby the demographics that are likely to use the VA services are more likely to be black, female, unmarried, and have little education for securing employment that has comprehensive health coverage. Boscarino et al. (2020) also indicate that upon returning from the war zone, veterans in rural areas report low VA service. However, PTSD, major depression, and alcohol addiction are significant issues that contribute to the severity of the veterans in rural settings. Still, marital status, education, age, and gender are among the factors contributing to the severity of these issues.

Mental health issues, especially among veterans, are critical issues that have created a dilemma for all other Americans. Hester (2017) found that 20% of the American population was uninsured for mental health services, and they primarily rely on public healthcare facilities and interventions for mental health crises. The American Mental Association veterans have experienced mental health crises since they returned from the warzone; issues such as depression, family issues, and alcoholism have become more common and increased. (Hester, 2017). An investigation was conducted to determine whether some soldiers entered the military with mental issues. The discovery was that attention deficit disorder (ADD) and explosive disorders were among the common mental issues that soldiers encountered in their early lives, and they later affected their social and economic lives. (Korpel et al., 2019). Mental disorders, especially from warzone events, including trauma, are predictors of suicidal thoughts and accidental mortality.

VA Health and US Veterans

The number of Americans who have deployed for military operations outside the United States has been increasing for the last two decades, raising concerns over the welfare of Veterans. Elnitsky et al. (2013) found that 2.3 million Americans have been deployed to Operation Enduring Freedom and Operation Iraqi Freedom (OEF-OIF) in the last two decades to combat the war crisis in Afghanistan or Iraq since 2002. It is essential to note that veterans participating in this (OEF-OIF) special operation are eligible to access VA healthcare services. However, the challenges these individuals have encountered have exceeded the cost coverage provided by the VA health system. (Elnitsky et al., 2013). Some of the issues that have been cited include the social pressures that result from mental stigma and the dread that they are burdening the system, as the primary barriers to accessing the desired health services. The focus of this case was to remove the barriers to mental health services, including mental health stigma, and to enhance the accessibility to healthcare from a personal point of need. (Mobbs & Bonanno, 2018). It was also vital to recognise that veterans have extended needs that may extend beyond the scope of VA health coverage. At the same time, the key advantages veterans enjoy concerning their utilisation of the VA are that it enhances the continuity of care while reducing the costs incurred while seeking these essential health services. The veterans encounter restrictions towards accessing VA exclusive care since two-thirds of the veterans have reported that they discovered barriers when seeking specific health interventions. (Elnitsky et al., 2013; Mobbs & Bonanno, 2018) As a result, the presence of obstacles predicted varying perspectives among veterans concerning the use of telehealth services, with barriers doubling the likelihood that war returnees would not exclusively use VA healthcare services.

One of the issues that increased the likelihood of veterans not using the VA health system was the geographical barriers. Davis et al. (2023) found that geographical distance significantly increased the possibility of veterans not utilising the VA healthcare services exclusively. One of the issues experienced was long wait times that doubled the likelihood of avoiding VA services. There are no evident disparities in the exclusive use of the VA services between the veterans identified to have polytrauma and the other returning military members. This further complicates the VA policies and frameworks regarding accessibility and care access.

Most veterans in the United States reside in rural areas. According to statistical information from the National Centre for Veterans Analysis and Statistics and the VA, approximately 4.4 million veterans live in remote residential areas of the United States, representing up to 42% (Amaral et al., 2018). Most veterans living in rural regions embrace the utilisation of VA healthcare, as 61% of the veterans who live in rural areas exclusively depend on VA healthcare services. (Finley et al., 2017)This population differs in the age composition of the individuals who access healthcare services. Most veterans who utilise VA healthcare are older adults, with 54% being 65 years or older. (Marshall et al., 2021). Among these, 54% of those residing and accessing rural VA healthcare, 60% have service-related conditions, and Black/American or Native Alaskan individuals were less likely to attend five or more sessions. (McKee et al., 2023). This makes the rural population the most vulnerable group of individuals who need the help of an enhanced healthcare system to address diverse needs.

Veterans in rural areas face similar challenges to those of other rural residents in accessing healthcare services. There are higher poverty rates in rural areas, which result in homelessness, mental disorders, and critical physiological health needs such as cochlear implantations. (Shayman et al., 2019). The health issues of the rural area residents are exacerbated due to the higher demand for mental health care and treatment, which is not readily available and is expensive to be insured by other healthcare systems. Substance use disorders have a close connection with the diverse experiences that veterans and poor populations in rural areas undergo. In most cases, alcohol and other substances, such as tobacco, are highly used in remote areas as a way of reducing the mental effects of stress, anxiety, and PTSD that veterans have experienced in missions and military operations. (Finley et al., 2017). It is vital to note that some veterans are unaware of the existing VA facilities that can be utilised to help facilitate critical health services. VA medical facilities have attempted to address the issues that veterans face in rural areas by establishing a framework that partners them with community health centres, Rural Health Clinics (RHCs), and hospitals. (Miller et al., 2021). These facilities can be as close as 10 miles apart and are more accessible than the VA healthcare system. At the same time, Telehealth and mobile VA clinics have developed approaches to bring healthcare services closer and more accessible to veterans in rural areas. (Day et al., 2021)The primary advantage of these initiatives is that they address the economic challenges faced by soldiers due to poverty and the lack of opportunities for veterans to transition from military to civilian life. The VA healthcare system depends on non-profit service organisations to bring services closer to veterans and enhance the uptake of these services to address personal health needs, more than mental healthcare. (Finley et al., 2017). The VA has also been keen on addressing the issues affecting rural veterans, primarily through programs like the Veteran Community Care Program, which offers healthcare services to veterans meeting the eligibility criteria from rural community providers.

There has been a significant change in the number of veterans accessing VA healthcare based on age, gender, race, and ethnicity. A longitudinal study conducted by Yoon et al. (2022) to investigate access to healthcare among veterans in five states found that 20 million enrolled for VA services across the United States. Five states — Arizona, California, Florida, New York, and Pennsylvania — are included, with the base year being 2012. The researchers focused on comparing the enrollment records, VA hospitalisation data, and discharge rates of VA beneficiaries (Yoon et al., 2022). While specific demographic characteristics, such as age, gender, ethnic background, and marital status, were considered, other more specific factors were found to influence access to VA healthcare. These include the VA enrollment category, community characteristics, and the date of death of the veterans from the time they enrolled for the services. The key findings from the research conducted by Yoon et al. (2022) revealed a significant increase in the number of veterans registered under the VA healthcare system, from 2.2 to 2.4 million, over a five-year period beginning in 2012. The percentage of men within this population of enrollees aged 61-62 years was 92-94%. This suggests that more men served as veterans compared to female veterans. At the same time, there was an increase in the number of people who sustained disabilities from the warzone from 24% to 33% (Yoon et al., 2022). However, there was a significant decline in veterans' hospitalisation over the five years. Acute hospitalisation decreased by about 14%, while VA community-funded hospitalisation increased by 26% (Yoon et al., 2022). In this case, the research confirms that a significant problem hindered accessibility to VA healthcare, especially for veterans, who anticipated community-level hospital facilities. Although Medicaid insured about 54% of the hospitalisations among veterans, it paid for an insignificant number (2%) of the hospital stays. (Zogg et al., 2019)These findings are justified by the fact that Medicaid was comprehensive enough to address the issues facing veterans.

Uniformity in the VA System

The service provision by VA healthcare has been found to raise concerns over its uniformity. Crowley et al. (2021) conducted a study investigating potential barriers to veteran healthcare, including the availability and extent of services, provider characteristics, and logistical approaches to delivering primary healthcare to veterans. Crowley et al. (2021) found that females experienced more structural barriers to healthcare. There were more barriers to accessing VA healthcare for women, as the services lacked uniformity, with some facilities offering services that were specifically tailored to women. In contrast, others integrated care into a more extensive system. The critical barrier in this case was a lack of sensitivity and competence, as the VA care providers failed to identify distinct services for women. (Crowley et al., 2021)Women's healthcare needs are different from those of men, and VA staff's perceived lack of sensitivity may hinder women's access to healthcare services. Although the VA has historically been involved in providing healthcare for more males than females, the lack of knowledge about women's veteran healthcare needs may hinder accessibility to quality services. (Marshall et al., 2021). A more uniform barrier to healthcare access by veterans is the logistical factors influenced by the physical environment, especially for veterans residing in remote and underserved areas.

Factors Limiting VA Accessibility

Several factors have been identified as limiting the availability of VA healthcare services. Segal et al. (2019) found that the geographical distribution of the VA facilities was among the most incredible challenges hindering the accessibility of healthcare services. Veterans and others with mobility challenges often face difficulties accessing VA healthcare due to the lengthy travel distances involved. In essence, the logistics of the services from the healthcare facilities positioned at different stations within the rural areas are far from the residential areas of the veterans. (Cyr et al., 2019). This is a common challenge faced by the general rural patient population, not just veterans. However, veterans have higher chances and vulnerability of experiencing at least one critical mental or physical healthcare concern. For instance, the prevalence of mental illness among veterans is more significant than among the general patient population in rural areas. (Segal et al., 2019) Numerous VA facilities are located in substantial metropolitan areas, posing a challenge for rural-based veterans in accessing prompt healthcare. In this case, the VA's eligibility requirement impedes the veterans' efforts to access healthcare.

The eligibility criteria for veterans are one significant barrier that has hindered access to the desired medical care. Segal et al. (2019) confirm that veterans who have been discharged for non-VA-acceptable reasons and those whose service terms are limited do not meet the eligibility criteria for receiving critical health services, such as mental health services. The resultant implication of this observation is the development of cognitive gaps whereby some can access VA healthcare services while others may not. The fundamental qualification for veterans to receive VA services is an honourable discharge from military service.

Additionally, the lack of mental healthcare and related services is another critical challenge to accessing mental healthcare. The research found that veterans pursuing mental health services had to wait longer for an appointment for their mental issues. (Rafferty et al., 2019). While mental issues are a growing concern for most veterans, the inconvenience caused in the process of service access has been found to significantly worsen the health condition of remote-based veterans who are in search of services. The combat veterans have a more significant concern for mental health, a concern that requires timely intervention.

Another cause of concern regarding the mental healthcare of veterans within the VA healthcare system is the substandard quality of care. Patel et al. (2020) found that while VA provides quality care for preventive care and management of chronic illnesses, disparities remain unaddressed by the healthcare system. The VA has shown diverse differences and disparities in the quality of care that it provides, primarily for veterans who live in rural and underserved areas. Veterans are at a higher risk of cardiovascular illnesses compared to non-veterans (Shukla et al., 2023). However, the quality of services for veterans has not improved, despite this critical observation. This highlights why veterans require prompt and timely care for the healthcare conditions they experience more than non-veterans. The inadequate access to quality care and disparities in who accesses certain services, and why, create a concern for veterans since this results in a higher risk of adverse health outcomes (Marshall et al., 2021). The disparities in quality healthcare can be attributed to challenges in healthcare delivery caused by underlying factors such as inadequate specialised staff to handle the increasing number of patients, a backlog of claims for health benefits among veterans, and the utilisation of outdated technology in healthcare, which leads to inefficiency. (Crowley et al., 2021). As a result, the veterans have experienced longer waiting times after booking appointments, leading to delays in receiving the required healthcare services. In some cases, the veterans may opt to seek private mental and physical health services, which are expensive.

The VA has faced budget constraints, which have limited its ability to expand the scope of healthcare service delivery throughout the system. Van Slyke and Armstrong (2020) found that, due to untimely medical intervention, the rural veteran population has faced significant challenges in receiving the required healthcare, primarily because the complexity of their conditions often exceeds the scope of rural VA healthcare systems. For the new patients seeking primary healthcare, the waiting times for diagnosis and treatment of complex health conditions such as cardiovascular, mental health, and physical disabilities have been a barrier. Research has indicated that patients experience challenges, especially in the wait times, which can be longer than 40 days, due to the lengthy procurement of healthcare services. (Govier et al., 2023). This not only creates barriers to the vulnerable veteran population but also increases the safety threats among the patients, leading to more health concerns.

Theories for the Study

Theories relevant to VA healthcare for veterans must address the social welfare of veterans and the suitability of the system in improving patient healthcare outcomes. Two theories are relevant for this research: social justice and system theory. These frameworks are suitable for this research as they enhance the understanding of the causes and factors that hinder veterans' access to healthcare through the VA healthcare system. (Jayasinghe et al., 2022). The social justice theory proposition holds that all community members have equal rights to access the social services, opportunities, and resources that benefit their social welfare. One of the fundamental social opportunities and resources is access to healthcare services regardless of gender, ethnic background, disability, culture, race, and identity. It is a violation of social justice, especially when the veterans cannot access fundamental health services due to the barriers that exist primarily in the scope of coverage for mental health services, diagnosis and treatment of disabilities sustained from war zone injuries, and disparities in the eligibility criteria for treatment of critical health conditions such as cardiovascular illnesses. (Marshall et al., 2021). Veterans and non-veterans should have access to high-quality healthcare services as long as they have accepted the obligation to serve their country. They form a significant part of American society, defending the ideologies that make America great, and their services need to be highly appreciated. The denial of healthcare services or complications in the procurement process, with delayed access and lengthy appointment procedures, hinder the accessibility of high-quality healthcare services. (Jayasinghe et al., 2022). The prevalence of mental illnesses among veterans can be attributed to the lack of a comprehensive framework to prioritise urgent matters that require immediate attention.

Social theory encompasses social services, including health, as well as the political and economic well-being of individuals. For instance, the political aspect affects workers' social welfare, as policies formulated by the government and local leaders often do not address their immediate needs. The allocation of economic resources depends on the political policies of those in power. The most significant financial issue that has worsened the health accessibility of the veterans is a constrained budget that does not prioritise offering high-quality services to veterans who served in the military, including comprehensive health coverage for chronic health conditions, disabilities and mental illnesses. The violation of social justice is a critical concern that hinders the support system that veterans are entitled to and the appreciation of the services that the veterans offer to the country.

On the contrary, systems theory is a distinct concept that provides a comprehensive understanding of how social work operates as a complex entity. A system is a simple framework to achieve a particular goal (Ungar, 2019). In other words, it functions as a whole through the interconnected parts of its individuals. Veterans' services are an example of a system in which individuals, organisations, families, and society cooperate to deliver or access specific services. The key concept that should be keenly analysed is that the solution cannot consider every part when discussing. Instead, every part is viewed as connected to others, whereby if there is a change in one entity, the system changes in the manner it operates. Systems theory applies to the VA healthcare system, whereby all organisations are viewed as a whole system and not treated as individual entities. The critical relevance of systems theory lies in the fact that the VA system comprises various components, including healthcare facilities, government-formulated policies, the funding framework, and medical personnel, all of which collectively influence veterans' access to healthcare services (Ungar, 2019). The emphasis of the systems theory in this research is to assess how each system structure works and how its change may affect the whole system. The eligibility of the VA and the standardised criteria, due to limited resources and budgetary constraints, have been found to affect veterans' access to services. Some of the requirements that affect veterans include the duration of their military service, the level of disability, and their income. While this criterion is discriminatory from an individual-level assessment, adjusting the evaluation of eligibility requirements, starting at the patient level, may impact the entire system (Crowley et al., 2021; Cyr et al., 2019). The government, for instance, may consider those who have been critically affected in terms of mental illness severity to be prioritised, meaning that more facilities and medical personnel will need to be deployed to handle the rising cases of mental illness. The budgetary allocation may also need to be balanced so that veterans in rural settings can access the same quality of services by bringing facilities closer to them, thereby sustaining service delivery. The overall result of this system adjustment is to reduce the number of veterans who are homeless on the streets, help them transition into civilian life, and encourage them to seek sustainable job opportunities that will enable them to support their families. Therefore, systems theory provides a straightforward approach to understanding how veterans' social work is interconnected with the VA healthcare system. Excursion can result in disparities in access to primary healthcare using the VA system, especially for low-income-earning veterans and the minority population, resulting in a precise interplay of the social justice and systems theory. Coordination and communication among these social entities require an understanding of power dynamics within the VA system, so that appropriate and more suitable services can be delivered to veterans.

Synthesis of Literature

The Veterans Affairs healthcare system is a comprehensive and complex framework focused on providing health services to millions of veterans across the United States. The veterans require critical and diverse healthcare due to the complexity of their combat operations, resulting in various health concerns. Among the healthcare needs that the veterans require is mental healthcare. This is the most significant concern for the veterans based on the traumatic and actual field operations that result in complicated mental illnesses such as post-traumatic stress disorder and depression. The combat operations have also been linked to other conditions that require special medical attention, including respiratory cancers, traumatic brain injuries, and musculoskeletal injuries. (Patel et al., 2020). This is true, especially in the combat operations in the Gulf and related states such as Iraq. Shukla et al. (2023) noted that the deployment of military personnel in places such as the Gulf has exposed the soldiers to dust and intense heat, smoke, and chemicals from explosives and firearms. These risks expose individuals to health risks during the deployment period. At the same time, accidents are expected during the deployment and combat military operations and can result in partial or permanent disability. Sustained injuries may affect various body parts, including the spinal cord, and affect the body's motor functions. These are severe health conditions that should be covered within the VA, yet there is no comprehensive framework that assesses the needs of such victims.

The veterans living in rural and underserved areas are more vulnerable to mental, psychological, and physical health conditions. Several factors have been identified as hindrances to accessing VA health services in remote areas. First, the economic welfare of rural veterans has not been adequately addressed. Most of them are poor, and they belong to the minority ethnic groups. As a result, accessing healthcare through the VA, which may be far from the residential areas, becomes a challenge. In this case, the challenge is not the availability of health services, but rather their accessibility. For instance, the nearest VA healthcare facility may be located as far as 1,000 miles away, which is a considerable distance that requires a reliable means of transportation to access the services. The poor veterans in the rural areas are, therefore, disadvantaged. The problem identified in this case is the gaps in the distribution of healthcare services across the rural population, ensuring that every Veteran has access to them.

Another issue that has been identified is the information gap on healthcare consumption among the veteran population. There is no clear distinction between the VA and non-VA customers, and the service planning policies are diverse and inclusive. Although economic planning and budget allocation are not significant challenges, making healthcare services more readily available is a significant challenge. A clear distinction has not been established to assess the differences in socioeconomic status and military services between the veterans who utilise VA healthcare and those who do not. The assessment at the individual level plays a critical role in developing a mechanism that groups veterans into service levels based on their socioeconomic, mental, and physical health. This perspective can be explained by the fact that some veterans do not seek mental health services due to stigmatisation, lack of financial resources to facilitate access, disabilities, and lack of support in transitioning from the military to everyday social life. These are among the critical underlying issues that have not been well comprehended.

Research Methodology

The methodology forms the fundamental part of research by connecting the problem statement, the questions, and objectives to the literature reviewed and the findings. The literature synthesis has already outlined that various challenges have not been addressed due to a lack of understanding of the gap in economic, social, and political welfare, as described by social justice and systems theories. The research methodology section identifies the data to be collected, which will answer the research questions and reveal the existing relationship between the VA healthcare systems and Veteran access to healthcare services. The VA system comprises individuals, organisations, families, and society as the fundamental parts that interplay to complete the system. The primary research method employed in this study is secondary data analysis from various sources to identify the factors that contribute to the complexity of the VA and why it struggles to address the diverse health needs of veterans on a personal level. The systematic examination of the data is vital in informing policies and decisions that can make VA healthcare sustainable across all dimensions. Some secondary data sources that may be appropriate include electronic health records, patient surveys, research journal articles, and other government databases that contain relevant information about the factors hindering veterans' comprehensive healthcare access using the VA system.

Although determining the reliability of secondary data analysis may be challenging, the validity of the information lies in studying as many sources as possible to ensure comprehensive understanding. The reason for preferring this method is that it offers data from the past ten years, enabling the researcher to develop an objective overview of the challenges that hinder the accessibility of healthcare services through the VA system. Secondary data analysis is also readily available, providing a more cost-effective method for conducting extensive research that can be applied to a broader scope of the veteran population. The cost-effectiveness does not limit the extent to which the researcher can work to unravel the natural complexities that hinder access to healthcare services for the veteran population, especially in remote areas of the United States. The recommendations from the secondary data analysis are related to the gaps identified from the literature review. This implies that the recommendations sections can be as dependable as possible.

Methods

The specific research method employed in this paper will involve a systematic review of the literature, including articles from online libraries and databases, as well as the Preferred Reporting Items for Systematic Reviews and Meta-Analyses (PRISMA). The method is dependable as it focuses on identifying sources, planning for data extraction, determining the information to be obtained from them, and assessing the relevance of the sources. In this manner, the researcher ensures that all sources meet the required guidelines for consistency and integrity in their review. The PRIMA guideline is also crucial in ensuring that the research is not arbitrary or biased when selecting the sources to be included in the study. (O'Dea et al., 2021). Since the analysis of secondary sources does not guarantee that the researcher will obtain the information they are seeking, decision-making in selecting sources is crucial for the researcher. In the PRISMA literature review procedures and guidelines, the readers can identify areas where the researcher was subjective in not adhering to the planned source extraction and analysis protocol. The systematic literature review, therefore, considers PRISMA guidelines as one of the approaches in secondary data analysis to make the research dependable and accurate.

Research Design

The research design for the secondary data analysis will involve both quantitative and qualitative aspects of data collection and analysis. Specifically, the qualitative data will be collected across four dimensions and will be descriptive, detailing the issues facing VA access and utilisation among rural veterans. In other words, the data collected will collect the views from different scholars and information written within articles to determine how these challenges in VA integration among rural veterans exist and the potential solutions to these obstacles. From the quantitative perspective, the data will be collected and analysed quantitatively in graphs and tables. In this manner, the challenges will be identified and grouped to produce an observable trend that can easily answer the research question in line with the study's objectives.

Sources of Data

The research will not focus on gathering first-hand information from interviews, case studies, or surveys, but rather on information that has already been obtained. As a result, secondary data will be accepted from reliable online libraries and websites, as well as systematic literature reviews and original research articles. Grey literature will also be obtained from other reliable sources, such as the World Health Organisation (WHO) and government websites, including the US Department of Veterans Affairs, if available. The best platform for conducting this research is the PubMed Cochrane Library, and the best platform that enables direct linkage to other reliable libraries is Google Scholar. Other platforms included were MEDLINE, ScienceDirect, and CINAHL. While access to information is unlimited, it will be crucial for the study to focus on sources that provide relevant information, including the most recent data, so that when the study makes recommendations, they will be more accurate and appropriate for improving healthcare access for soldiers. All sources must be published within the last ten years and written in English. Keywords, especially those related to the topic, problem, and research questions, will be entered into the search engine to retrieve a variety of sources to be included in this study. The reference lists of the sources relevant to the survey were searched, and entries were made.

Search strategy

The strategy for this research was to identify the most relevant sources that would be most suitable in a fundamental sense. The literature search used CINAHL, Google Scholar, PubMed, ScienceDirect, and Cochrane as the primary websites, libraries, and databases. The justification was to find as many sources as possible to include within the study, but the inclusion criteria had to be met. Some of the keywords to be included were challenges and barriers to the VA healthcare system, rural veterans, rural quality of care, barriers to veterans' access to healthcare, economic challenges in VA healthcare access, potential solutions to VA healthcare barriers and challenges, mental health for rural veterans, diversification of VA healthcare for women, and challenges to specialty care among the rural veterans. The keywords were combined to create longer sentences and words that would maximise the scope of the sources, ensuring the research would utilise a variety of sources. The Boolean operators "AND" and" OR" were primarily utilised to enhance access to various sources, exposing the researcher to diverse opinions for data analysis to generalise the findings. For instance, the operator "OR" combined phrases like rural veterans OR VA barriers, potential solutions OR VA healthcare challenges, and special care OR diversification. "AND" was also found to have significant applicability in maximising the research results, and some of the appropriate combinations included (rural veterans AND quality healthcare, economic challenges AND diversification of VA healthcare, and challenges to VA access and Solutions). The results of this search strategy increase the likelihood of finding the most reliable and relevant sources published within the last ten years. Although combining words using Boolean operators was employed, a different approach was taken to identify relevant literature, particularly from the WHO website. The platform also enhanced comprehension of specific trends, statistical relationships, and key terminologies used across diverse dimensions. The primary reason for utilising information from WHO is to support the existing literature, incorporating findings from articles and grey literature, allowing for a comparison during data analysis to identify further gaps or detect any unreliability that may impact the research.

Removal of duplicates

Removing duplicate sources is crucial to minimise inconvenience, as the article may be available on multiple platforms. The reference lists must also be managed to ensure they do not reappear. Some sources from databases such as Google Scholar and the WHO website may contain the same author and year of publication. Mendeley Desktop managed the bibliographic information to ensure it was correctly listed by removing duplicates and creating a distinction between sources. The citations of the different articles will be inserted within the paper so that the final lists of the sources that will be generated do not comprise duplicate sources.

Inclusion and Exclusion Criteria

The inclusion and exclusion criteria for the sources form another critical aspect that cannot be ignored, as the research aims to be reliable and valid, despite its focus on secondary data analysis. The inclusion and exclusion criteria fall into four major categories: the year and relevance of the research questions and objectives, the quality of articles and their reliability, the comprehensiveness of the sources and study populations, and the specific outcomes or findings of the research.

***Table 3.* Inclusion and exclusion criteria**

Criteria	**Inclusion**	**Exclusion**	**Rationale**
Year and Relevance to Research Questions and Objectives.	The source must have been published within the last ten years and directly contain aspects the research questions seek	Published before the last ten years, and does not contain data that directly answers the questions.	Due to the need to obtain the most current and relevant data about veterans' access to VA healthcare.

	to answer.		

The Quality of Sources and the Reliability	Sources must contain systematic reviews of the original research approaches. The websites could also contain grey data published by reliable organisations such as	Case reports and case series	Research needs to obtain reliable, systematically researched, and synthesised data. These would be indicators and tools for gathering information that have been used in studies.

	the WHO, government websites, Case-control studies, qualitative studies, and other tool development articles.		

Study Populations and Comprehensiveness	The articles must contain comprehensive data about the veteran population and the VA healthcare system.	Generalised findings about patients.	The data sources should be relevant only to veterans and the VA healthcare system.

Outcomes	Reports VA quality indicators and tools for veterans' healthcare quality, barriers, challenges, and solutions.	Does not report VA quality indicators and tools for veterans' healthcare quality, barriers, challenges, and solutions.	The reason is to answer the questions and achieve the objectives of this research.

Data extraction

The data regarding the barriers and challenges to VA healthcare access were extracted. The indicators were categorised into four dimensions (geographical disparities between the urban, suburban, and rural settings, the immediate healthcare need based on diversity, patterns, VA utilisation, and actual challenges). The categorisation of the data into these dimensions considered the significance of the research questions and objectives that had already been established. The extraction of data using this framework was to ease analysis and synthesis.

Data synthesis

After the research extracted data, it was grouped into the four selected indicators: geographical immediate care needs and how veterans utilise them. Based on the synthesis of the information, the research aimed to develop the necessary recommendations, which are among the core objectives of this research paper.

Results

The literature search yielded ten sources, as illustrated in Figure 1. These sources met the inclusion criteria based on the framework provided in Table 1. The sources that met the requirements were then comprehensively involved in the study.

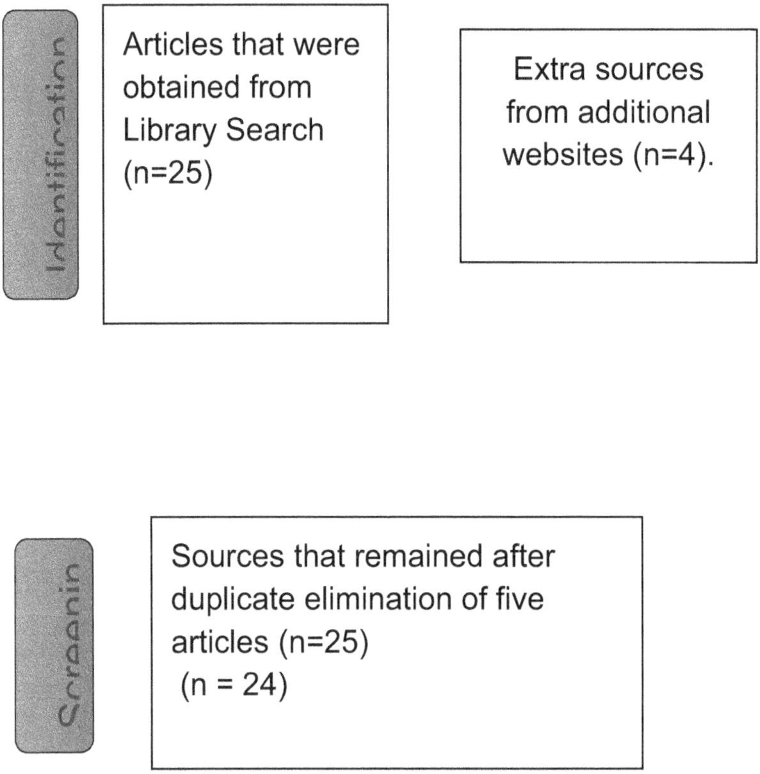

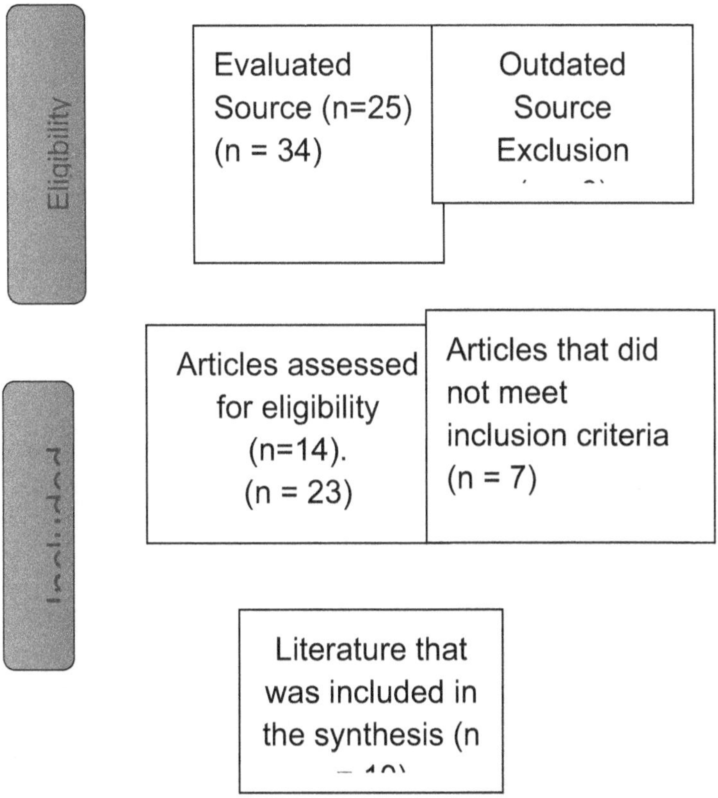

Figure 3. PRISMA Diagram for Data Source Search Assessment and Entry

tudy	Geographical Disparities	Healthcare Needs	VA Healthcare Utilisation Patterns	Challenges and Barriers
Cyr et al., 2019)	The geographical distribution of behavioural health professionals in rural areas was only 1/3 of that in urban centres.	1. ealth screening for underlying conditions 2. ubstance abuse treatment services, 3. pecial care and treatment ,	Rural Wisconsin and Utah veterans showed significantly lower utilisation of VA healthcare than urban residents. The utilisation rates of rural-based veterans	- ender and culture affected the perceptions about telehealth integration. - vailability and accommodation of

		including surgeries	were 17% lower than those of urban veterans.	special health needs were challen ging for most vetera ns. - elayed screeni ng for up to 30 days - overty
Teich et al., 2017)	Th e geograph ic distance between	Me ntal Health Treatmen t	The rural-based patients were 70% less likely	- Physic al health status

	residential areas and healthcare facilities poses a significant challenge. There were fewer VA healthcare facilities in rural areas than in urban areas.	Prescriptions for mental health treatment.	to access mental health services. The rural veterans were 52% less likely to access mental health outpatient services and 64% less likely to receive prescriptions.	- Unemployment and low-income distribution in rural areas - Low education levels - Higher severity of psychiatric disorders in rural areas

Gurewich et al., 2021)	The greater geographic distance was observed as the main challenge.	Physical therapy Cardiology tests and procedures Optometry Orthopaedic	Rural veterans have consistently relied more on non-VHA healthcare than their urban counterparts. 20.7% of rural veterans prefer Community Care (CC) compared to those in urban centres, where only 11%	- elayed access to the VA healthcare services - istance barriers - ome of the available VHA hospitals were closed. - hortage of special

			Physical therapy had an average wait time of about 28 days, while optometry and orthopaedic services exceeded 30 days.	ists and healthcare providers.
Butkus et al., 2020)	There was no substantial discussion of the geographical distance	Injuries and deaths from firearms Treatment of the environmental hazards	The current statistics indicate that opioid use disorders have affected the ethnic minorities	- Stigma affects healthcare access for racial minorities

	as a factor.	Treatment of substance use disorders	in rural Alaska more than those living in urban centres.	- Workforce shortage in rural areas affects the quality of healthcare delivery.
Slightam et al., 2020)	The geographical distance was an issue in accessing VA	Accessibility to specialised care. Mental health condition	The rural population has the lowest telehealth usage, at 25%, compared	- Lack of knowledge among the rural-based

	healthcare The travel was found to be greater	s found to be chronic include PTSD, depression, and hypertension.	to the urban veteran population, at 61%. Prevalent health conditions among the rural populations include hypertension at 51.6% and depression at 50.9%. While PTSD was the most common, it was prevalent	veterans. Digital gadgets, such as tablets, were not available and affordable among the rural veteran population. - Willingness to engag

			in the rural population at 45.5%.	e with the care providers. A lack of training and support hindered access to virtual VA services.
Derefinko et al., 2019)	-	Mental health issues such as PTSD	The veterans report higher rates of suicide	- Strained family relationship

		and suicidal thoughts. Re adjustment support Ec onomic welfare through employment Ch allenges in accessing diverse healthcare needs.	due to mental health issues at 21% compared to 16% of civilians who do not access mental health services. 70% of veterans who did not access the VA healthcare system committed suicide.	- Economic and financial challenges and homelessness - Challenges in transitioning from military to civilian life. - Inaccessibility

				of mental healthcare services, such as therapy
Dallocchio, 2021)	-	Mental health access Specialised health services for women	Women veterans, especially ethnic minorities, have experienced challenges to quality healthcare access.	- Disparities when it comes to ethnic minority weapons. - The systemic pattern

				of marginalising women of colour and other vulnerable social groups has hindered intersectionality. - Women have been retraumatised in

				the process of reintegrating into society. - Stigma towards veteran women - Lack of trained personnel to deal with diverse populations,

				embrace equity and Inclusion - Institutionalised discrimination
Chang et al., 2020)	-	Special care for Mental healthcare for high-risk veterans was the primary healthcare.	High-risk veterans are among the smallest portion of veterans whose healthcare needs are more costly than	- High cost of special care and hospitalisation for high-risk specialists.

		Vulnerable conditions, such as spinal cord injuries, necessitated access to exceptional VA healthcare. Substance use disorder therapy was among the primary health services	those of others. While the high-risk veterans were fewer, 88% were assigned general primary healthcare. High-risk veterans utilised the in-person, telephone, and secure messaging platforms to access exceptiona	- Inadequate specialised personnel for high-risk cases. Old veterans, as they grow older, often acquire a disability. Distance becom

		that veterans were searching for.	l healthcare.	es an issue for some patients who require specialised care.
Rasmussen & Farmer, 2023)	Rural veterans have challenges of distance, which go beyond the eligibility requirements for	The services accessed include surgeries, chronic health conditions, and mental health.	Rural veterans' healthcare needs are higher than average compared to those in urban areas. VA-eligible veterans	The Veterans Health Administration (VHA) focuses on eligibility criteria

	VA services.		can pay for non-VA community healthcare, although the providers are not affiliated with the VA. Most rural veterans prefer VA healthcare providers to those in urban areas.	for access to healthcare. The eligibility criteria hinder service access because it depends on when the military service commenced, the period

				served, the conditions that led to discharge, and service-related issues such as sexual trauma and disability.
US Department of	Rural-based veterans are more affected	-	-	Disability rating, income

Veterans Affairs, 2024)	by the eligibility criteria than their urban counterparts.			level, and military service history are the primary factors considered when accessing VA healthcare.

Table 4. Data collection from individual eligible sources in four dimensions

Data Analysis

The data from the ten sources will be analysed, considering the facts related to the four dimensions. The data obtained has been categorised into four dimensions and visual representations. An individual source analysis will be conducted to ensure the reliability and consistency of the authors' statements from the sources and their relevance to the research findings.

From the ten sources, it is evident that from the first source by Cyr et al. (2019), the geographical distribution of behavioral health professionals in rural areas was only 1/3 of that in urban centres, whereby the Health screening for underlying conditions of substance abuse treatment services, and special care and treatment, including surgeries, were the significant health needs of the patients in the rural areas. Although this situation is typical for all veterans, the rural-based veterans highly depend on the VA healthcare to access healthcare services. Based on the trend in telehealth utilisation in a comparative model, rural Wisconsin and Utah veterans showed significantly lower VA healthcare utilisation patterns compared to urban residents. This is the only instance where the rural VA utilisation was lower in rural than urban centres.

In other words, all the remaining eight articles, except the last, indicate that the dependency on VA health is higher in rural areas than in urban areas. Some of the barriers and challenges that could contribute to the VA not meeting its goals among the veteran populations include poverty, unemployment, gender, and culture, which affect the perceptions about telehealth integration. Availability and accommodation of special health needs were a challenge to most veterans, while the accessibility challenge was mostly delayed screening for up to 30 days. The physical health status and low-income distribution in rural areas resulted in high dependency yet low access to the available VA healthcare systems, which were less evenly distributed in remote settings than in rural areas.

Table 3 below presents a breakdown of the information gathered from the analysis of secondary sources in four dimensions. From the data obtained, the approximate distribution of the most significant dimension influencing VA access among veterans has been presented in a graph in Figure 2 below.

Table 5. Analytical Distribution of Dimensions influencing VA accessibility

Analytical Dimension	Geographical Disparities	Healthcare Needs	A Healthcare Utilisation Patterns	Challenges and Barriers
Number of Issues identified	7	24	9	35

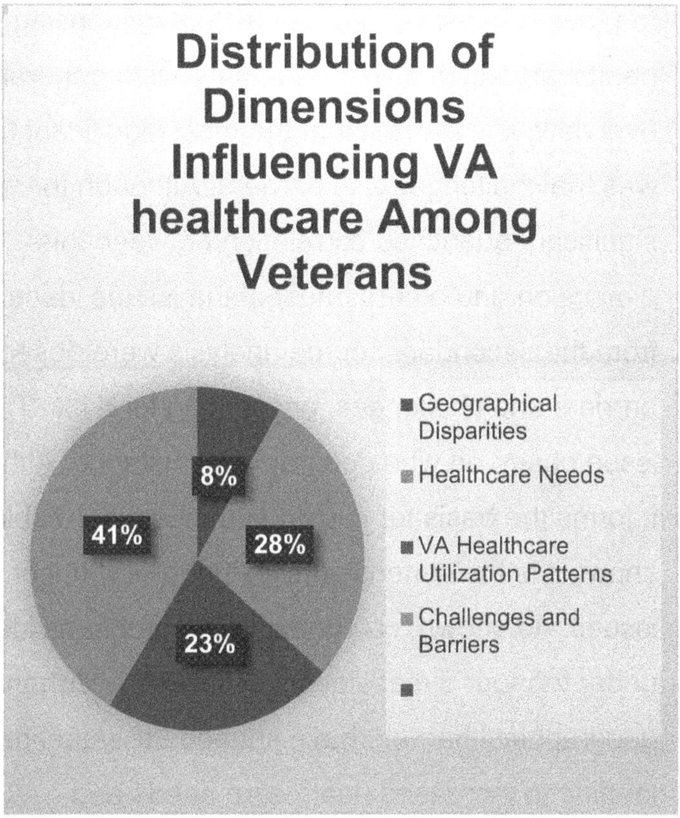

Figure 4. The Graphical Presentation of Dimensions Influencing VA Healthcare Among Veterans

Figure 2 shows a correlation between the four dimensions and the factors influencing healthcare access. While the figure is a generalised overview, it is evident that the most significant factor was the challenges and barriers. Although there is no significant quantified correlation between this dimension and others, most of the issues identified from the secondary source analysis were observed as barriers and challenges, accounting for 41%. The only issue observed was geographical distance. Although it forms the basis for causing other issues, Table 2 shows it is the dimension with the fewest minor issues. As shown, categorising the problems identified under the four dimensions justifies the notion that geographical barriers have shaped utilisation patterns, leading to increased healthcare needs and challenges. This is the only justifiable relationship between the four dimensions and their analytical perspective.

Results

Three sources cite that education levels significantly hinder access to quality and desirable healthcare services. Seven of the ten sources mention a challenge with healthcare accessibility. Distance accessibility and an economic perspective suggest a closer relationship between VA challenges and healthcare quality. Although the services were available in some instances, special care was unavailable, as most sources indicate based on the four dimensions of data acquisition.

About three sources have cited social aspects such as discrimination, inequality, strained family relationships, and stigma as challenges to accessing the VA healthcare system. Two sources indicate that technological issues were more common among the rural veteran population. The eligibility criteria are a significant factor hindering access to healthcare, but the sources have not adequately addressed them.

Findings of the Empirical Study

Several findings justify the existence of barriers and challenges to VA healthcare access, as well as the precise ways in which they manifest. Some of these obstacles can be addressed without engaging economic resources, but through carefully analysing the gaps identified throughout the research.

Qualitative Themes

Among the sources associated with geographical disparities identified as among the most significant challenges are 7 out of the ten sources. This represents 70% of the sources that indicated geographical issues. One of the sources suggests that the geographical distribution of behavioural health professionals in rural areas was only 1/3 of that in urban centres. This implies that the distribution issue hinders access to healthcare through the VA system. The geographic distance from residential areas to healthcare facilities is a significant challenge, resulting in economic constraints for economically challenged rural veteran residents. In the fourth source, the geographical distribution of VA healthcare facilities in rural areas was found to be less than in urban areas. There is a more significant correlation between geographical distance, availability, and demand for healthcare services. Although no clear relationship was established between distance and uptake, rural veterans demanded VA healthcare more frequently than urban-based residents. In the fifth source, the travel distance was associated with the travel cost, introducing an issue of efficient and timely access to health services at the convenience of veteran patients. In addition to geographic location, rural veterans preferred to settle in remote areas, as some did not meet the eligibility criteria.

The healthcare needs represent another vital theme about the diversity of healthcare services demanded under the VA health system. Each of the sources indicated different healthcare needs. However, the most common healthcare needs were substance abuse and mental health treatment services. All the sources revealed that the primary issue affecting accessibility to the VA was mental healthcare, which depended on the eligibility of the veterans. The first source found that health screening for underlying conditions, substance abuse treatment services, and special care and treatment, including surgeries, are needed. The second source was more specific in highlighting the challenges faced by healthcare practitioners, including physical therapy, cardiology tests and procedures, as well as optometry and orthopaedic treatment services. From the third source, the healthcare needs were more severe. They required special care, which has been cited as a challenge related to delayed access to VA healthcare services and the closure of the available VHA hospitals. At the same time, the diverse healthcare needs required special care, which was hindered by the barriers of a lack of specialised care, yet there were fewer unique care providers.

Still on the healthcare needs, there was the need for healthcare services across rural veterans for services, including the injuries sustained from firearms. The environmental hazards, such as intense heat from the sun and dust, required special treatment services, which were unavailable to the rural populations. However, there is no clear relationship between the healthcare needs and the barriers to achieving the treatment goals due to factors like stigma among racial minorities and a shortage of workforce in rural areas, affecting the quality of healthcare delivery. The healthcare needs identified under the mental health category for the fifth source include PTSD, depression, and hypertension. These healthcare needs are directly related to a lack of knowledge among rural-based veterans and inadequate access to digital gadgets such as tablets. They were not available and affordable among the rural veteran population. The willingness to engage with the care providers and lack of training and support affected virtual VA access and also worsened the treatment of issues like PTSD. The sixth source justifies that mental health issues, such as PTSD, resulted in suicidal thoughts due to challenges in readjustment to everyday civilian life. The economic difficulties affected the veterans' transition to civilian life, presenting challenges in accessing employment and seeking and settling into income-generating opportunities outside of military life.

Quantitative Themes

The quantitative results are also critical to the data analysis and the generation of results that will answer the questions identified from the background theory. Table 3 presents the diverse patient needs and the number of patients requiring healthcare services, as extracted from research data on high-risk veterans conducted by Chang and colleagues. The results are presented in Figure 3, which shows the pattern and trend of VA health utilisation among high-risk veterans. From the identified qualitative themes, high-risk veterans most frequently utilised general health services. This represents the highest number of veteran patients needing special care. At the same time, it is evident that the most readily available services cater to general health needs, including minor surgeries, health assessments, and general prescriptions. These are believed to be less costly and do not require special care. When considering the challenges that led to the observations in Figure 3, two factors can be identified as the underlying issues related to these observations. First, the high cost of special care and hospitalisation for high-risk specialists hinders the accessibility of special health services. The second challenge is the inadequate availability of specialised personnel for high-risk cases. In this context, the high-risk patients require highly specialised care. The most significant reason is the

Special care for Mental healthcare for high-risk veterans was the primary healthcare. Vulnerable conditions, such as spinal cord injuries, necessitated access to exceptional VA healthcare.

Substance use disorder therapy was among the primary health services that veterans were searching for. High-risk veterans are among the smallest portion of veterans whose healthcare needs are more costly than those of others.

While the high-risk veterans were fewer, 88% were assigned general primary healthcare.

High-risk veterans utilised the in-person, telephone, and secure messaging platforms to access exceptional healthcare.

Table 6. Diverse Patient Service Needs

Veteran Patient Service Category	**Number of patients**
General Healthcare Seekers	308 433
Diverse Women's Healthcare Needs	15885
Geriatrics	6447
Homeless Veterans	2775
Home-Based Primary Care	8139
Other Special Healthcare Needs	9333

Figure 3 was obtained from the table above. The figure below provides several insights concerning the accessibility of specialised veteran services. The highest distribution of veterans seeking healthcare lies among general healthcare seekers. These individuals seek regular health services for normal conditions since the illnesses are manageable and not chronic.

The VA system offers these services because they are cheaper, and most veterans are eligible to access them.

Interpretation of Results

Women veterans have experienced more challenges in accessing VA healthcare services that satisfy their needs. Although they form the second-highest figure of the patient population requiring exceptional healthcare, the critical factor to consider is that the VA has not been established to be inclusive regarding gender. The barriers justify the findings, such as the high cost of special care and hospitalisation for high-risk specialists and inadequate specialised personnel for high-risk cases. Diversified healthcare services for veteran women require more specialised care under the VA system. Still, there are no clear guidelines and frameworks that enhance the accessibility of these services. The VA system is complicated due to the high number of veterans who have been served over the past two decades and the constrained budget to deliver healthcare services, depending on the services offered to the United States by the veterans.

While Figure two offers a general overview, the barriers identified by source 6 are more definite in providing the reason women are among the high-risk veterans. The source notes that institutional marginalisation is among the factors that affect not only women but also the minority members of society. There have been disparities when it comes to ethnic minority welfare in VA and non-VA healthcare. Issues such as systemic patterns of marginalising women of colour and other vulnerable social groups have hindered intersectionality, leading to low access to the desired health outcomes among high-risk veterans. When comparing the risk exposure between men and women veterans, women are at a higher risk of either not accessing health care or facing unique and diverse health challenges. The sixth source explicitly mentions that women have been retraumatised in reintegrating into society. Although their service delivery might be the same as that of men and eligibility criteria are constant, veteran women encounter challenges such as marginalisation against their expectations that they would receive equal health services just as men. Men experience societal barriers such as stigma. Still, there has been greater stigmatisation against women, a challenge that results in more women opting to either seek non-VA healthcare or shy away from accessing the required health services.

The last issue that has been associated with low access rates among women and other ethnic minorities from the research findings is the lack of trained personnel to deal with diverse populations and embrace equity and Inclusion. People of colour and other ethnic minorities have additional social challenges in terms of institutionalised discrimination. This critical issue that leads to all these barriers is institutionalised discrimination.

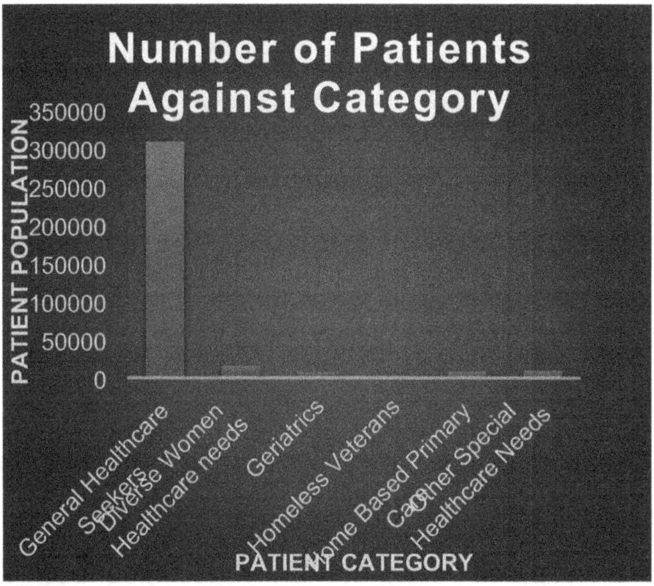

Figure 5. Distribution of Service Access Among the High-Risk Veterans

Geriatrics is a unique population that the VA healthcare system considers essential to the patient population. However, these individuals from Figure 3 form an insignificant portion of high-risk veterans who have minimal access to primary healthcare services. These individuals comprise approximately 3% of the total veteran population in VA healthcare. While there is no clear correlation between low accessibility and old age, several factors are associated with older adults not accessing the required healthcare services using the VA healthcare system. Although most of them are covered by Medicare, older veterans have been found to shift from the VA to non-VA healthcare significantly. Some of the reasons for the low accessibility, as indicated in the figure above, are the increasing medical complexity of the old veterans as they grow older and the acquisition of disability. As a result, travelling to facilities far away from their residential areas poses a challenge to older adults. This justifies why some older adults are seeking specialised and general care. In the urban centres, there are competing healthcare facilities, both Veteran and non-veteran, including exceptional hospitals, which are preferred by high-risk veterans, including those with spinal injuries and those seeking special care, such as HIV patients. These results indicate a low number of older patients seeking VA-specialised healthcare.

Homeless veterans have raised a severe contention over social institutions and healthcare facilities regarding the factors that lead to homelessness and how they influence the quality of care for veterans. This is among the serious issues the research has found, considering that this population has the lowest access to the VA healthcare system. Regarding the challenges and barriers, Table 2 presents a range of issues that have influenced healthcare access, particularly for rural-based veterans. The data obtained indicates that physical health status, unemployment, low-income distribution in rural areas, low education levels, and higher severity of psychiatric disorders in rural regions hinder access to healthcare. These issues reveal a complex relationship, but in this study, the significant issues were the geographical distance and distribution of services in rural regions. This insight addresses R1, which aims to identify the challenges and barriers to VA healthcare access for rural veterans. While other problems, such as poverty, contribute to inadequate access to healthcare services, homelessness can be attributed to poverty, economic constraints, and low education levels, which are more prevalent in rural areas.

Additionally, the trend in telehealth utilisation has been significantly associated with poverty, homelessness, and low-income distribution in rural areas. For instance, rural Wisconsin and Utah veterans showed significantly lower utilisation of VA healthcare than urban residents. The utilisation rates of rural-based veterans were 17% lower than those of urban veterans. In addition to this, rural-based patients were 70% less likely to access mental health services. The rural veterans were 52% less likely to access mental health outpatient services and 64% less likely to receive prescriptions. From these observations, it is evident that rural-based veterans face more challenges than their urban-based counterparts. At the same time, the utilisation patterns indicate that most rural veterans prefer Community Care (CC) over those in urban centres. The justification for this observation is linked to the geographical distance experienced by the veterans.

Rural veterans have consistently relied more on VHA healthcare than their urban counterparts. The current statistics indicate that opioid use disorders have affected the ethnic minorities in rural Alaska more than those living in urban centres. Drug and substance usage from the literature review has been identified as the most significant challenge hindering mental health access. The literature review still confirms that mental health issues are most prevalent among veterans, and they have resulted in disorders such as PTSD and depression. The usage of drugs and substances, including alcohol, not only puts the veterans into poverty but also results in substance use disorder. This results in complications of family relationships between the veterans and their loved ones. Although there is no clear relationship between family relationships and homelessness, the complex interaction between drug usage disorders, economic challenges, and addiction in rural areas results in homelessness. This worsens the health status of rural veterans, making them more vulnerable to critical conditions such as mental disorders and other health conditions.

The rural population has the lowest telehealth usage compared to the urban veteran population. High-risk veterans utilised the in-person, telephone, and secure messaging platforms to access exceptional healthcare. These primary healthcare approaches have been found to address the distance and limit the availability of healthcare facilities in rural areas. Most rural veterans prefer VA providers to community-based healthcare providers due to the complexity of mental and physical illnesses. At the same time, high-risk veterans are among the smallest portion of veterans whose healthcare needs are more costly than those of others, yet they form the majority of the population living in rural areas. While PTSD was the most common high-risk mental illness among veterans, it was prevalent in the rural population. The veterans report higher rates of suicide due to mental health issues that are not addressed in time, due to delayed medical accessibility and critical health interventions. Prevalent health conditions among the rural populations include hypertension and depression.

Conclusion and Recommendations

Several conclusions have been drawn from the research based on the research questions. Rural-based veterans have more critical and risky health conditions that require specialised care. However, these services are mostly not available in rural areas.

Veterans primarily rely on VHA facilities, which often have a complex procurement process in rural areas.

Major Conclusions

The most significant challenge identified in the analysed data was the inaccessibility of quality health services, especially for veterans, due to geographical distance and social disparities. Women veterans, especially ethnic minorities, have experienced challenges to quality healthcare access. While the high-risk veterans were fewer, they were assigned general primary healthcare, which did not meet their health outcomes, considering that primary healthcare services among rural veterans are critical. The data collected indicate that the healthcare needs of rural-based veterans are higher than those of the average urban population. At the same time, they face the most significant barriers of distance, poverty, and economic neglect.

For the first research question, which seeks to determine the challenges and barriers to VA healthcare access for rural veterans, several challenges have been identified as disproportionately affecting rural-based residents compared to urban and suburban populations. The availability and accommodation of special health needs in rural settings were a challenge to most veterans. Although a few of these services, primarily for the high-risk veterans, were available, delayed screening and diagnosis of chronic illnesses such as cardiovascular and physical injuries sustained from firearms and weapons affected the rural veterans, and they also affected the urban populations. In this context, the eligibility criteria hinder service access because it depends on when the military service commenced, the period served, conditions that led to discharge, and service-related issues such as sexual trauma and disability, as outlined by the VA system. The assessment of eligibility criteria among rural veterans was delayed by factors such as distance and challenges in travelling to reach the few facilities distributed in rural areas.

Due to constrained resources, the VHA must consider veterans' eligibility based on their rating disability, income level, and military service history, which are the fundamental aspects considered before accessing VA healthcare. For instance, some veterans who served in the military long enough to complete the specified missions may be eligible for services due to the successful execution of these missions, such as those in Afghanistan and the Gulf wars. The research, however, did not investigate how the history of military service would influence eligibility. However, an honourable discharge from the military may allow the veterans to access various services offered within the VHA. VA-eligible veterans can pay for non-VA community healthcare, although the providers are not affiliated with the VA.

In addition to the unavailability of VA services in rural areas, another barrier is the closure of some available VHA hospitals. Although the critical challenge from this perspective is the lack of the required services despite the availability of the VA facilities, rural veterans still prefer the VA. However, alternative community healthcare facilities were available. This addresses the second research question, which aimed to identify the challenges and barriers to VA healthcare access that impact the quality and well-being of veterans. The delayed diagnosis and treatment of high-risk conditions, such as physical disabilities sustained from the combat operation and mental illnesses, resulted in other medical conditions, such as the development of suicidal thoughts. These issues required more diversified care.

On the other hand, the social aspect has been related to hindering the accessibility of healthcare in rural settings. Some of these barriers include gender and culture affecting perceptions about telehealth integration, stigma that influences healthcare access to racial minorities, and discrimination against specific minority veteran populations residing in rural areas due to poverty and economic constraints. These factors influenced the willingness to engage with the care providers, especially among the rural veterans who were mainly affected by the social and institutional marginalisation issues. Challenges in transitioning from military to civilian life have been cited in secondary sources, but they are more commonly associated with the general problems soldiers face. However, some of the veterans required services such as counselling services that would enable them to transition from the military to social life. In this case, disparities when it comes to ethnic minority health service delivery were not only a challenge but a factor that affected access to quality healthcare through the VA system. The systemic pattern of marginalising women of colour and other vulnerable social groups has hindered the diversification of services and the development of a comprehensive healthcare system that would include even the needs of minority social service providers. The specific challenge has been the retraumatisation of women as they struggle to reintegrate into society.

Lastly, the lack of knowledge among rural-based veterans affected access to healthcare delivery in rural populations in several ways. First, inadequate education limits access to better employment opportunities, especially in the private sector, where particular skills and attitudes are required. Essentially, the difficulty in transitioning from Veteran to civilian life was challenging since the soldiers could not quickly settle into civilian life, and this could be related to inadequate education among the veteran population. Lack of training and support has affected virtual VA access to healthcare, as the rural population lacks adequate knowledge to utilise the telehealth services that aim to reduce distance barriers.

Recommendations Based on the Results

Potential solutions to the barriers and challenges of utilising the VA system can be addressed through several approaches. Most of these recommendations are designed to promote the long-term sustainability of rural healthcare through the VA system. One of the most significant challenges is distance barriers due to the lack of healthcare facilities in rural settings. This challenge can be resolved through expanding telehealth coverage in rural areas. This is a potential solution to the geographical barriers, which are the underlying cause of most economic and social barriers. However, telehealth should be improved because it offers patient-centred services by assessing the health needs of soldiers who need general primary healthcare.

For the high-risk veterans who have issues with mobility, the mentally ill, and the soldiers who have sustained chronic injuries, it would be vital to offer transportation assistance. This should not be limited to those who have special health needs, such as the mentally ill and those who sustained injuries during combat operations, but also to the economically challenged who cannot afford the transportation cost to move from their residential areas to the VA healthcare facilities. In this context, it is vital to note that the veterans prefer VA healthcare to community-based care.

Community healthcare providers could also coordinate with the VA healthcare system in rural areas to bridge the gaps in accessibility. For instance, if the healthcare needs are not critical and require highly specialised personnel, veterans can visit nearby facilities to access the same level of services. The shortage of healthcare professionals can be addressed by motivating healthcare providers through incentives, enabling them to engage more with rural-based veterans.

For the second research question, health education initiatives can be implemented among rural veterans to enhance access to specialised healthcare services. Since mental health is among the issues hindering access to healthcare among veterans, it would be critical to offer mental health support to the veterans so that there is self-awareness that military life is different from social life. Peer support programs can substitute individualised special care. The VA system should partner with community-based facilities and organisations to identify the issues that should be prioritised among the veterans and establish ways to solve emerging problems, such as seeking employment opportunities through skills development to alleviate poverty.

The timely access to VA healthcare is relevant to research question R3. Due to accessibility issues, the VA should invest in mobile clinics to provide diverse healthcare services at the community level, rather than relying on patients to visit specific facilities. While virtual care has been hindered by poverty and economic constraints, it should be among the plans that the VA should prioritise specifically for veterans in rural areas to provide them with gadgets that can enhance virtual communication and diagnosis. The last but not least approach is to diversify technological integration in VA healthcare, so that patients with high-risk conditions, such as cardiovascular conditions, can be assessed and reached within a short time.

Summary

In summary, access to primary healthcare through the VA system is a crucial aspect that should be considered when evaluating the importance of veteran services to the American public. The research has identified several challenges that have influenced and hindered veterans' access to quality care, especially those in remote regions. Substance use disorder therapy was among the primary health services that veterans have prioritised for mental health conditions such as PTSD. High-risk veterans are among the smallest portion of veterans whose healthcare needs are more costly than those of others, and this is the reason their services are unique. Diversified healthcare services for veteran women require more specialised care under the VA system. Still, there are no clear guidelines and frameworks that enhance the accessibility of these services. While there is no clear correlation between low accessibility and old age, several factors are associated with older adults not accessing the required healthcare services using the VA healthcare system. Homeless veterans have raised a severe contention over social institutions and healthcare facilities regarding the factors that lead to homelessness and how they influence the quality of care for the veterans. The rural population has the lowest telehealth usage compared to the urban veteran population. High-risk veterans utilised the in-person, telephone, and secure messaging platforms. The research methodology and design involved secondary data analysis, using the PRISMA approach to select the relevant findings.

In conclusion, improving primary healthcare involves addressing geographical barriers by utilising telehealth, community healthcare coordination, assisting veterans with transportation, and employing more community healthcare providers. However, the research was limited by factors such as the analysis of secondary sources, the division of the issues influencing healthcare access into four dimensions, and the enhancement of access and availability of healthcare services. Based on the research findings, recommendations for further research focus on enhancing inclusivity and revising eligibility criteria to make more services accessible to a broader range of patients.

References

Amaral, E. F. L., Pollard, M. S., Mendelsohn, J., & Cefalu, M. (2018). Current and Future Demographics of the Veteran Population, 2014–2024. *Population Review*, *57*(1). https://doi.org/10.1353/prv.2018.0002

Ayele, R. A., Liu, W., Rohs, C., McCreight, M., Mayberry, A., Sjoberg, H., Kelley, L., Glasgow, R. E., Rabin, B. A., & Battaglia, C. (2021). The VA Care Coordination Program Increased Primary Care Visits and Improved Transitional Care for Veterans' Non-VA Hospital Discharge. *American Journal of Medical Quality*, *36*(4), 221–228. https://doi.org/10.1177/1062860620946362

Boscarino, J. J., Figley, C. R., Adams, R. E., Urosevich, T. G., Kirchner, H. L., & Boscarino, J. A. (2020). Mental health status in veterans residing in rural versus non-rural areas: the Veterans' Health Study results. *Military Medical Research*, *7*(1), 44. https://doi.org/10.1186/s40779-020-00272-6

Butkus, R., Rapp, K., Cooney, T. G., & Engel, L. S. (2020). Envisioning a Better U.S. Health Care System for All: Reducing Barriers to Care and Addressing Social Determinants of Health. *Annals of*

Internal Medicine, *172*(2_Supplement), S50. https://doi.org/10.7326/M19-2410

Chang, E. T., Zulman, D. M., Nelson, K. M., Rosland, A.-M., Ganz, D. A., Fihn, S. D., Piegari, R., & Rubenstein, L. V. (2020). Use of General Primary Care, Specialised Primary Care, and Other Veterans Affairs Services Among High-Risk Veterans. *JAMA Network Open*, *3*(6), e208120. https://doi.org/10.1001/jamanetworkopen.2020.8120

Cheney, A. M., Koenig, C. J., Miller, C. J., Zamora, K., Wright, P., Stanley, R., Fortney, J., Burgess, J. F., & Pyne, J. M. (2018). Veteran-centred barriers to VA mental healthcare services use. *BMC Health Services Research*, *18*(1), 591. https://doi.org/10.1186/s12913-018-3346-9

Crowley, R., Atiq, O., Hilden, D., & Cooney, T. G. (2021). Health Care for Our Nation's Veterans: A Policy Paper From the American College of Physicians. *Annals of Internal Medicine*, *174*(11), 1600–1602. https://doi.org/10.7326/M21-2392

Cyr, M. E., Etchin, A. G., Guthrie, B. J., & Benneyan, J. C. (2019). Access to speciality healthcare in urban versus rural US populations: a systematic literature review. *BMC Health Services Research*, *19*(1), 974. https://doi.org/10.1186/s12913-

019-4815-5

Dallocchio, M. (2021). Women Veterans: Examining identity through an intersectional lens. *Journal of Military, Veteran and Family Health*, *7*(s1), 111–121. https://doi.org/10.3138/jmvfh-2021-0028

Davis, M., Snider, M. J. E., Hunt, K. J., Medunjanin, D., Neelon, B., & Maa, A. Y. (2023). Geographic variation in diabetic retinopathy screening within the Veterans Health Administration. *Primary Care Diabetes*, *17*(5), 429–435. https://doi.org/10.1016/j.pcd.2023.06.004

Day, S. C., Day, G., Keller, M., Touchett, H., Amspoker, A. B., Martin, L., & Lindsay, J. A. (2021). Personalised implementation of video telehealth for rural veterans (PIVOT-R). *MHealth*, *7*, 24–24. https://doi.org/10.21037/mhealth.2020.03.02

Derefinko, K. J., Hallsell, T. A., Isaacs, M. B., Colvin, L. W., Salgado Garcia, F. I., & Bursac, Z. (2019). Perceived Needs of Veterans Transitioning from the Military to Civilian Life. *The Journal of Behavioural Health Services & Research*, *46*(3), 384–398. https://doi.org/10.1007/s11414-018-9633-8

Elnitsky, C. A., Andresen, E. M., Clark, M. E., McGarity, S., Hall, C. G., & Kerns, R. D. (2013). Access to the US Department of Veterans Affairs health system: self-reported barriers to care among returnees of Operations Enduring Freedom and Iraqi Freedom. *BMC Health Services Research*, *13*(1), 498. https://doi.org/10.1186/1472-6963-13-498

Finley, E. P., Mader, M., Bollinger, M. J., Haro, E. K., Garcia, H. A., Huynh, A. K., Pugh, J. A., & Pugh, M. J. (2017). Characteristics Associated With Utilisation of VA and Non-VA Care Among Iraq and Afghanistan Veterans With Post-Traumatic Stress Disorder. *Military Medicine*, *182*(11), e1892–e1903. https://doi.org/10.7205/MILMED-D-17-00074

Govier, D. J., Hickok, A., Edwards, S. T., Weaver, F. M., Gordon, H., Niederhausen, M., & Hynes, D. M. (2023). Early Impact of VA MISSION Act Implementation on Primary Care Appointment Wait Time. *Journal of General Internal Medicine*, *38*(4), 889–897. https://doi.org/10.1007/s11606-022-07800-1

Gurewich, D., Shwartz, M., Beilstein-Wedel, E., Davila, H., & Rosen, A. K. (2021). Did Access to Care Improve Since Passage of the Veterans Choice Act? *Medical Care*, *59*(Suppl 3), S270–S278. https://doi.org/10.1097/MLR.0000000000001490

Hester, R. D. (2017). Lack of access to mental health services contributes to the high suicide rates among veterans. *International Journal of Mental*

Health Systems, *11*(1), 47. https://doi.org/10.1186/s13033-017-0154-2

Hunt, M. G., Cuddeback, G. S., Bromley, E., Bradford, D. W., & Hoff, R. A. (2019). Changing Rates of Mental Health Disorders Among Veterans Treated in the VHA During Troop Drawdown, 2007–2013. *Community Mental Health Journal*, *55*(7), 1120–1124. https://doi.org/10.1007/s10597-019-00437-1

Jayasinghe, S., Faghy, M. A., & Hills, A. P. (2022). Social Justice and Equity in Healthy Living Medicine: An International Perspective. *Progress in Cardiovascular Diseases*, *71*, 64–68. https://doi.org/10.1016/j.pcad.2022.04.008

Jones, C., Miguel-Cruz, A., Smith-MacDonald, L., Cruikshank, E., Baghoori, D., Kaur Chohan, A., Laidlaw, A., White, A., Cao, B., Agyapong, V., Burback, L., Winkler, O., Sevigny, P. R., Dennett, L., Ferguson-Pell, M., Greenshaw, A., & Brémault-Phillips, S. (2020). Virtual Trauma-Focused Therapy for Military Members, Veterans, and Public Safety Personnel With Posttraumatic Stress Injury: Systematic Scoping Review. *JMIR MHealth and UHealth*, *8*(9), e22079. https://doi.org/10.2196/22079

Korpel, P. O. J., Varkevisser, T., Hoppenbrouwers, S. S., Van Honk, J., & Geuze, E.

(2019). The Predictive Value of Early-Life Trauma, Psychopathy, and the Testosterone–Cortisol Ratio for Impulsive Aggression Problems in Veterans. *Chronic Stress*, *3*, 247054701987190. https://doi.org/10.1177/2470547019871901

Marshall, V., Stryczek, K. C., Haverhals, L., Young, J., Au, D. H., Ho, P. M., Kaboli, P. J., Kirsh, S., & Sayre, G. (2021). The Focus They Deserve: Improving Women Veterans' Health Care Access. *Women's Health Issues*, *31*(4), 399–407. https://doi.org/10.1016/j.whi.2020.12.011

McKee, G. B., Knopp, K., Glynn, S. M., & McDonald, S. D. (2023). VA family service access and utilisation in a national sample of veterans. *Psychological Services*, *20*(3), 609–621. https://doi.org/10.1037/ser0000626

Meffert, B. N., Morabito, D. M., Sawicki, D. A., Hausman, C., Southwick, S. M., Pietrzak, R. H., & Heinz, A. J. (2019). US Veterans Who Do and Do Not Utilise Veterans Affairs Health Care Services: Demographic, Military, Medical, and Psychosocial Characteristics. *The Primary Care Companion for CNS Disorders*, *21*(1), 26992. https://doi.org/10.4088/PCC.18M02350

Miller, K. E. M., Miller, K. L., Knocke, K., Pink,

G. H., Holmes, G. M., & Kaufman, B. G. (2021). Access to outpatient services in rural communities changes after a hospital closure. *Health Services Research*, *56*(5), 788–801. https://doi.org/10.1111/1475-6773.13694

Mobbs, M. C., & Bonanno, G. A. (2018). Beyond war and PTSD: The crucial role of transition stress in the lives of military veterans. *Clinical Psychology Review*, *59*, 137–144. https://doi.org/10.1016/j.cpr.2017.11.007

O'Dea, R. E., Lagisz, M., Jennions, M. D., Koricheva, J., Noble, D. W. A., Parker, T. H., Gurevitch, J., Page, M. J., Stewart, G., Moher, D., & Nakagawa, S. (2021). Preferred reporting items for systematic reviews and meta-analyses in ecology and evolutionary biology: a <scp>PRISMA</scp> extension. *Biological Reviews*, *96*(5), 1695–1722. https://doi.org/10.1111/brv.12721

Ofori, W. A. (2020). *Impact of Socioeconomic Factors on U. S. Veterans' Access to Care*. ProQuest. https://www.proquest.com/openview/3cb1f155fe5c0cbd2c96831ff025d7a9/1?pq-origsite=gscholar&cbl=51922&diss=y

Patel, M. I., Lopez, A. M., Blackstock, W., Reeder-Hayes, K., Moushey, E. A., Phillips, J., & Tap,

W. (2020). Cancer Disparities and Health Equity: A Policy Statement From the American Society of Clinical Oncology. *Journal of Clinical Oncology*, *38*(29), 3439–3448. https://doi.org/10.1200/JCO.20.00642

Peterson, K., Anderson, J., Boundy, E., Ferguson, L., McCleery, E., & Waldrip, K. (2018). Mortality Disparities in Racial/Ethnic Minority Groups in the Veterans Health Administration: An Evidence Review and Map. *American Journal of Public Health*, *108*(3), e1–e11. https://doi.org/10.2105/AJPH.2017.304246

Rafferty, L. A., Wessely, S., Stevelink, S. A. M., & Greenberg, N. (2019). The journey to professional mental health support: a qualitative exploration of the barriers and facilitators impacting military veterans' engagement with mental health treatment. *European Journal of Psychotraumatology*, *10*(1). https://doi.org/10.1080/20008198.2019.1700613

Rasmussen, P., & Farmer, C. M. (2023). The Promise and Challenges of VA Community Care: Veterans' Issues in Focus. *Rand Health Quarterly*, *10*(3), 9. http://www.ncbi.nlm.nih.gov/pubmed/37333666

Segal, A. G., Rodriguez, K. L., Shea, J. A.,

Hruska, K. L., Walker, L., & Groeneveld, P. W. (2019). Quality and Value of Health Care in the Veterans Health Administration: A Qualitative Study. *Journal of the American Heart Association*, *8*(9). https://doi.org/10.1161/JAHA.118.011672

Shayman, C. S., Ha, Y.-M., Raz, Y., & Hullar, T. E. (2019). Geographic Disparities in US Veterans' Access to Cochlear Implant Care Within the Veterans Health Administration System. *JAMA Otolaryngology–Head & Neck Surgery*, *145*(10), 889. https://doi.org/10.1001/jamaoto.2019.1918

Shukla, S., Mbingwa, G., Khanna, S., Dalal, J., Sankhyan, D., Malik, A., & Badhwar, N. (2023). Environment and health hazards due to military metal pollution: A review. *Environmental Nanotechnology, Monitoring & Management*, *20*, 100857. https://doi.org/10.1016/j.enmm.2023.100857

Slightam, C., Gregory, A. J., Hu, J., Jacobs, J., Gurmessa, T., Kimerling, R., Blonigen, D., & Zulman, D. M. (2020). Patient Perceptions of Video Visits Using Veterans Affairs Telehealth Tablets: Survey Study. *Journal of Medical Internet Research*, *22*(4), e15682. https://doi.org/10.2196/15682

Teich, J., Ali, M. M., Lynch, S., & Mutter, R. (2017). Utilisation of Mental Health Services by

Veterans Living in Rural Areas. *The Journal of Rural Health*, *33*(3), 297–304. https://doi.org/10.1111/jrh.12221

Ungar, M. (2019). Designing resilience research: Using multiple methods to investigate risk exposure, promotive and protective processes, and contextually relevant outcomes for children and youth. *Child Abuse & Neglect*, *96*, 104098. https://doi.org/10.1016/j.chiabu.2019.104098

US Department of Veterans Affairs. (2024). *Eligibility for VA health care*. US Department of Veterans Affairs. https://www.va.gov/health-care/eligibility/

Van Slyke, R. D., & Armstrong, N. J. (2020). Communities Serve: A Systematic Review of Need Assessments on U.S. Veteran and Military-Connected Populations. *Armed Forces & Society*, *46*(4), 564–594. https://doi.org/10.1177/0095327X19845030

Yoon, J., Kizer, K. W., Ong, M. K., Zhang, Y., Vanneman, M. E., Chow, A., & Phibbs, C. S. (2022). Health Care Access Expansions and Use of Veterans Affairs and Other Hospitals by Veterans. *JAMA Health Forum*, *3*(6), e221409. https://doi.org/10.1001/jamahealthforum.2022.1409

Zogg, C. K., Scott, J. W., Metcalfe, D., Gluck,

A. R., Curfman, G. D., Davis, K. A., Dimick, J. B., & Haider, A. H. (2019). Association of Medicaid Expansion With Access to Rehabilitative Care in Adult Trauma Patients. *JAMA Surgery*, *154*(5), 402. https://doi.org/10.1001/jamasurg.2018.5177

Chapter 9

Nursing Q & A

Content

When a pulse is present, how often should rescue breaths be given in infants and children? One breath every 2 to 3 seconds.

Priority Decision: Triage the following patient situations that may be present in an emergency department (ED) as 1, 2, 3, 4, or 5 on the Emergency Severity Index.

Patient Situation 1: 35-year-old male presenting with chest pain and diaphoresis

- Triage Level: ESI 2

Patient Situation 2: 28-year-old woman with a severe asthma exacerbation, speaking in one-word sentences and using accessory muscles to breathe

- Triage Level: ESI 1

Patient Situation 3: 50-year-old man with acute abdominal pain radiating to the back, vomiting, and diaphoresis

- Triage Level: ESI 2

Patient Situation 4: 67-year-old woman with a cough, fever, and body aches for two days

- Triage Level: ESI 4

Patient Situation 5: 25-year-old man with a laceration to the hand after cutting himself with a kitchen knife, controlled bleeding

- Triage Level: ESI 5

When a nurse performs a primary survey in the ED, what is she assessing?

A - Airway with Cervical Spine Protection

B - Breathing

C - Circulation with Haemorrhage Control

Disability (Neurological Status)

E - Exposure/Environmental Control

Additional Considerations in the Primary Survey

When a pulse is present, how often should rescue breaths be given in infants and children? One breath every 2 to 3 seconds.

In Basic Life Support (BLS), rescue breathing is a critical intervention for infants and children when a pulse is present, but they are not breathing or breathing inadequately. The rate of rescue breaths when a pulse is present differs for infants and children compared to adults. The American Heart Association (AHA) guidelines recommend administering one breath every 2 to 3 seconds, translating to approximately 20 to 30 breaths per minute.

The difference in timing between infants, children, and adults is due to their distinct physiological needs. Children and infants have a faster respiratory rate and a higher metabolic demand than adults, so they require a more frequent supply of oxygen to meet their bodies' needs. If they are not breathing adequately but have a pulse, prompt and correctly timed rescue breaths help oxygenate their tissues, preventing hypoxia and other severe complications.

To ensure effectiveness, the person delivering rescue breaths should follow proper technique:

1. Airway positioning: Ensure the airway is open by tilting the head and lifting the chin (in infants, this is done more carefully to avoid overextension of the neck).

2. Seal and breaths: Provide breaths using either a face mask or a barrier device. If no barrier device is available, mouth-to-mouth or mouth-to-nose (for infants) can be used. Provide each breath over 1 second and ensure a visible chest rise.

3. Monitoring: Continue rescue breaths while monitoring the child’s pulse. If the pulse is absent or falls below 60 beats per minute despite effective rescue breaths, start chest compressions, as this is a sign of impending cardiac arrest.

Frequent re-evaluation of the child's respiratory and circulatory status is crucial, and rescue breaths should continue until the child begins to breathe adequately on their own or when professional medical help arrives. It is essential to recognise the signs of respiratory failure or deterioration in children and infants, as they often show subtle signs before progressing to complete respiratory arrest.

Priority Decision:

Triage the following patient situations that may be present in an emergency department (ED) as 1, 2, 3, 4, or 5 on the Emergency Severity Index.

The Emergency Severity Index (ESI) is a triage system used in emergency departments to prioritise patient care based on the severity of their condition. It uses a five-level scale, with ESI 1 being the most critical (requiring immediate life-saving interventions) and ESI 5 being the least urgent. Each patient scenario is prioritised from 1 to 5 based on their presentation and the anticipated resource need.

Here is the triage for each patient situation using the ESI:

Patient Situation 1: 35-year-old male presenting with chest pain and diaphoresis.

- **Triage Level: ESI 2**

This patient is presenting with symptoms consistent with a potential myocardial infarction (heart attack), including chest pain and diaphoresis (sweating). Although the patient is not in immediate cardiac or respiratory arrest (which would be ESI 1), they are at high risk for serious complications such as cardiac arrest or other life-threatening conditions if not treated promptly. Therefore, this patient should be triaged as **ESI 2**, which requires rapid evaluation and treatment to prevent deterioration.

Patient Situation 2: 28-year-old woman with a severe asthma exacerbation, speaking in one-word sentences and using accessory muscles to breathe.

- **Triage Level: ESI 1**

This patient is experiencing a severe asthma attack characterised by the inability to speak in complete sentences and the use of accessory muscles for breathing. These are signs of imminent respiratory failure, and the patient requires immediate intervention to secure the airway and improve oxygenation. Given the critical nature of her condition and the need for immediate life-saving intervention, this patient should be triaged as ESI 1.

Patient Situation 3: 50-year-old man with acute abdominal pain radiating to the back, vomiting, and diaphoresis.

- **Triage Level: ESI 2**

Acute abdominal pain, especially when radiating to the back and accompanied by vomiting and diaphoresis, can indicate a life-threatening condition such as a ruptured abdominal aortic aneurysm or severe pancreatitis. While this patient may not need immediate life-saving interventions at the moment of presentation, they are at high risk for rapid deterioration. This presentation warrants an ESI 2 triage level, requiring prompt evaluation and diagnostics to rule out severe conditions.

Patient Situation 4: 67-year-old woman with a cough, fever, and body aches for two days

- **Triage Level: ESI 4**

According to the patient's symptoms, an upper respiratory infection or influenza is most likely the cause of their viral respiratory sickness. Although uncomfortable, there is no imminent risk to life from the symptoms, and more than one resource is unlikely to be needed for a diagnosis or course of therapy.

The patient is in a stable general condition; however, further testing (e.g., a flu test or a chest X-ray) may be required to rule out potential complications, such as pneumonia. Consequently, this patient has to be a priority ESI 4.

Patient Situation 5: 25-year-old man with a laceration to the hand after cutting himself with a kitchen knife, controlled bleeding

- **Triage Level: ESI 5**

The bleeding from this patient's hand laceration is under control. Since the injury is minimal, there is no imminent risk to life or limb. Although therapy is required, it is likely to be limited to straightforward measures, such as cleansing the wound, suturing, or applying a bandage. The patient does not need many resources, and the damage has not affected their overall level of stability. An ESI 5 triage level is, therefore, appropriate in this case.

Summary of Triage Levels

1. ESI 1: Requires immediate life-saving intervention, as seen in the 28-year-old woman with a severe asthma exacerbation.

2. ESI 2: High-risk situations requiring prompt care but not immediately life-threatening, such as the 35-year-old male with chest pain and the 50-year-old male with acute abdominal pain.

3. ESI 3: Typically involves multiple resources, such as imaging or lab work, but the patient is stable.

4. ESI 4: Requires limited resources, such as a 67-year-old woman with a cough and fever.

5. ESI 5: Requires minimal resources, with injuries or conditions that are not immediately life-threatening, as in the 25-year-old man with a hand laceration.

In conclusion, triaging patients in an emergency department is a dynamic and critical process that ensures that those needing immediate care receive it while allocating resources efficiently. Using the ESI system helps emergency personnel quickly identify the severity of conditions and prioritise patients based on the urgency of their situation.

When a nurse performs a primary survey in the ED, what is she assessing?

A primary survey in the Emergency Department (ED) is a systematic and rapid assessment conducted by a nurse to identify and manage life-threatening conditions. This assessment typically follows the ABCDE approach, which stands for Airway, Breathing, Circulation, Disability, and Exposure. Each element is assessed in the following manner:

A - Airway with Cervical Spine Protection

- The nurse ensures that the patient's airway is open and free from obstructions. It includes checking for visible obstructions, such as vomitus, foreign objects, or swelling, that may compromise breathing.
- At the same time, the nurse maintains cervical spine immobilisation to protect the patient from further injury, especially in trauma cases.
- Signs of airway compromise include stridor, hoarseness, gurgling, and inability to speak.
- Immediate interventions such as the chin-lift or jaw-thrust manoeuvres may be required, along with suctioning or inserting an airway device if needed.

B - Breathing

- The nurse evaluates the patient's breathing by assessing respiratory rate, depth, and effort. Symmetry of chest wall movement, breath sounds, and the use of accessory muscles are also noted.

- Using a stethoscope, the nurse listens to lung sounds to check for abnormal findings such as wheezing, crackles, or diminished breath sounds.
- Oxygen saturation is monitored using a pulse oximeter, and the nurse provides supplemental oxygen if necessary.
- Conditions that could compromise breathing include pneumothorax, haemothorax, or flail chest.

C - Circulation with Haemorrhage Control

- Circulation assessment focuses on evaluating the patient's cardiovascular status. It includes checking heart rate, blood pressure, pulse quality, skin colour, and capillary refill.
- The nurse palpates peripheral pulses to assess perfusion. Weak or absent pulses, hypotension, or signs of shock indicate compromised circulation.
- The nurse also examines the patient for signs of external bleeding and controls any haemorrhage with direct pressure or a tourniquet.

- Intravenous access is established, and fluid resuscitation or blood transfusions may be initiated.

D - Disability (Neurological Status)

- The nurse performs a quick neurological assessment using the AVPU scale (Alert, Verbal, Painful stimuli, Unresponsive) or the Glasgow Coma Scale (GCS) to evaluate the patient's level of consciousness.
- Pupillary response to light, limb movement, and signs of any focal neurological deficits are also assessed.
- Early identification of altered mental status, such as confusion or decreased consciousness, is critical for detecting potential head injuries or other neurological conditions.

E - Exposure/Environmental Control

- The nurse exposes the patient by removing clothing to conduct a complete visual assessment of the body for injuries, such as lacerations, burns, or fractures.
- This step ensures that no hidden injuries are missed.

- Simultaneously, the nurse maintains the patient's body temperature by providing blankets or warming devices to prevent hypothermia, which can exacerbate shock.

Additional Considerations in the Primary Survey

- The nurse may use adjuncts like pulse oximetry, electrocardiography (ECG), or blood glucose testing as part of the initial assessment.
- If any life-threatening issues are identified, immediate interventions are prioritised.

The primary survey aims to identify and address any immediate threats to life in a structured and timely manner, ensuring that critical conditions are not missed.

Author Qualifications and Honours

D.D., Doctor of Divinity

Certificate in Bible studies

Theology

Laws

(LLM)Master of Laws.

Postgraduate Laws

legal research,

Business, CSR, Corporate social responsibility and human rights law."

Institutional development and management,

International Law.

BA (Hons), Laws

Law: includes Criminal, Tort, damages, Contract, Property, Equity and Trust, European Law, Public, Constitutional, Judicial Review, and Agency.

Advance Dip. Business Law, Level 4: Employment, Agency, Damages, Tort, Contract, employment tribunal, etc.

Dip. Criminology

Accounting

BA (Hons)op.

Financial Accountant

Management Accountant

Cert. Acct. (Certified accountant)

(PCA)Professional Certificate in Financial and Management Accounting

Dip. Book-keeping, Level 3

Nursing

Nursing: RMN Registered Mental Nurse)

GN (General Trained Nurse)

Lecturer qualifications

DD Doctor of Divinity

LLM Master of Laws

BA (Hons)

BSc Hons o/g) Psychology with counselling

Cert. in Education (Lecturer)

Business Certificate in Advanced Management

Cert. Business Enterprise

Advanced Food Hygiene

Intermediate Health and Safety

Dip. Safety Management

International Entrepreneur for over 25 years

(NVQ); Internal Verifier, (V1)

Trainer and Assessor A1 (NVQ)

Computers

Diploma: Cisco Level 2 Technician (build, repair, networking)

Microsoft Specialist

Dip. Claire Plus (in all software)

New Clait Dip. Level 2

ECDL Level 2

Scrip writer

Diploma in script writing.

TV, radio, stage, and film

Diploma in writing.

Autobiography

Biography

Family History

Certificate in Poetry

Psychology and Counselling

BSc(Hons o/g) psychology with counselling

Diploma in Counselling and Psychology

Cert. in Counselling and Psychology

Certificate in Social Science

Photography

Cert. (PGFP).

Portrait, Glamour and Figure

Plumbing

Level 3 City and Guild

Hypnotherapy

Dip. Hypnotherapy

Other Books by the Author James Safo

162 book Titles.

Academic, Faith and non-faith books

Faith books- in 5 different languages :

Arabic, Chinese, English, French, Spanish

ALL FAITHS

Theology

Love All Faiths

Faith Unity

Religion and Law: Religion influences National and international laws.

CHRISTIANITY

BIBLE New Testament; 1,111 QUESTIONS AND ANSWERS: Plus, synopsis and Test yourself

Bible Old Testament 1,064 Questions and Answers and Synopsis

Jesus Christ is Coming Soon

God Loves Christianity

God's/Allah's Messengers

Islam v. Christianity

Jesus Christ is coming soon

Psychology of religion, politics and marriage

Faith unity.

Faith Unity Simplified Version.

Islamism versus Christianity.

Love all faith.

ISLAM (In English)

QUR'AN; 1,044 Questions & Answers.

Allah Loves Islam

Islam v. Christianity

BUDDHISM (In English)

God Enlighten Buddhism

HINDUISM (In English)

Parama Nandra Loves Hindus

FREEMASON (In English)

In Search of Wisdom in Freemasonry

FRENCH BOOKS (Religious)

Allah Aimel'islam (Allah loves Islam)

Aimetouteslesfois (Love All Faiths)

Islamism. V. christianisme (Islam v Christianity)

Dieu Aime Le Christianisme (God loves Christianity)

DISEASES Volume 1 J.Safo

Les Messagers De Dieu/ Allah (God/Allah Messengers)

A LA Recherche De La Sagesse Dans La Franc - Maconnerie (In Search of wisdom)

SPANISH BOOKS (Religious)

En Busca De La Sabiduria Masoneri (In search of wisdom in freemasonry)

Ametodas las creencias (Love All Faith)

Mensajeros de Dios (God Messengers)

4Dios Ama El Christianismo (God Loves Christianity)

Islam vs Christianity (Islam vs Christianity)

Allah am el Islam (Allah Loves Islam)

ARABIC (Religious)

الله يحب الاسلام. (Allah loves Islam) .

حب جميع الأديان Love All Faith .

DISEASES Volume 1   J.Safo

CHINESE BOOKS (Religious)

Books in Chinese

伊斯蘭教訴基督教 (Islam vs. Christianity)

上帝爱伊斯兰教 (Allah Loves Islam) - Traditional

Chinese Edition

NON-FAITH BOOKS- IN ENGLISH LANGUAGE

LAW:

Global Injustice

The Journey to Law Graduation

THE JOURNEY TO MASTER OF LAWS

International Laws plus 30 dissertation

Laws - United Kingdom +30 dissertation

The Law (Over 1,160 Questions and Answers)

Business Law volume 1; over 800 Q&A (contract, employment, types of Human Rights

Business Law Volume 2 over 600 Q&A (Tort, CSR, Equity, Trust

Criminology: (Over 1,300 Questions and Answers)

Religion And Law

POEMS

102 Poems on North America

DISEASES Volume 1 J.Safo

70 Poems on South American Countries and Cities

80 POEMS ON THE ARCTIC AND ANTARCTICA

102 POEMS ON AUSTRALIA, OCEANIA, NEW ZEALAND

101 Poems on Asia countries and cities

118 USA POEMS: 50 States, Cities and Maps

114 Poems on 54 African countries

Over 200 Love Poems plus over 100 love icebreakers

Over 100 Poems on Faith & Victory

107 Poems on Discrimination, Racism & Suffering

Jesus Christ, Prophet, Arch Angels, Saint (Over 150 poems and Biography

The One - Over 130 Poems "DCF"

105 Poems on 54 European Countries & Cities

BUSINESS

Developing and Managing Institutions and Organisations Volume 1

Developing and Managing Institutions and Organisations Volume 2

Set up and manage a business

How to set up a care home and care agency

How to manage a care home and a care agency

Care Home: Staff training

DISEASES Volume 1 J.Safo

COMPUTER

Computing for beginners + 310 questions and answers.

How to Build and Upgrade a Computer and Network

The Path of Information to the Computer Screen

Computer Programming, Coding & Science Dissertation

ACCOUNT

Financial Accounting (Over 1,241 Questions and Answers)

Management Accounting (1015 Questions & Answers Plus 100 Self-Assessment Questions)

PSYCHOLOGY

Journey to Psychology Graduation Volume 1

Journey to Psychology Graduation Volume 2

Psychology of Religion, Politics & Marriage

COUNSELLING

Journey to Counselling Graduation Volume 1

Journey to Counselling Graduation Volume 2

Counselling: Journey to Graduation Volume 3

Mood Disorder & Therapy

HISTORY

History: Journey to Graduation: 38 Essays

ENEMIES Within the Earth

Slavery And Suffering

Slavery to Mastership

GEOGRAPHY

Geography: The Road to Graduation: 30 Essays

Medical/Nursing/ Health & Social

Drugs for Diseases: 1,007 Questions and Answers

Health and Social Care

Journey to Nursing Graduation: 51 Essays

Mental and Physical Diseases - Plus Nursing and 53 Dissertations

Health and Social Care - Plus 50 Dissertations

SOCIAL SCIENCE

Understanding Sociology Science - Plus 56 Dissertations

WOMEN

Women are superior to men

Sweet and Sour Women (plus over 500 love letters from women)

MANAGEMENT

Project management

RESEARCH

Research

Midwifery

A modern approach to Agriculture, Introduction level,

Added Value to Agriculture: Advanced Level.

The Roadmap to Sustainable Agriculture in Rural Development.

The beekeeper's blueprint: growing your apiary from the ground up

Addictive Manufacturing

Quantity Survey

Building and Construction

Drug and Substance Abuse Rehabilitation

Education Volume 1 and 2

Radiology

Mental health V1,2, and 3

Geography Physical

Geography of Africa

Geography Techniques

Glossary (Medical)

A

Abdomen

The tummy area from the lower ribs to the pelvis.

Abortion;

Ending a pregnancy using either medicines (medical abortion) or an operation (surgical abortion).

Acute;

Sudden and severe.

Adenomyosis Endometriosis in the muscle wall of the uterus.

Adhesions;

Scars that connect two or more body structures.

Amniocentesis;

A way of testing the fluid surrounding a baby in the womb by taking a small sample with a needle inserted through the abdomen. It can be carried out after the 15th week of pregnancy, and can detect some conditions, like Down syndrome.

Amniotic fluid ;

The watery liquid surrounding and protecting the growing fetus in the uterus.

Amniotic sac;

The pregnancy sac contains the baby and the amniotic fluid. It is sometimes also called "the membranes".

Anaemia;

It is A condition where the level of haemoglobin, the protein in blood which carries oxygen around the body, is lower than usual. It can be mild or severe and may cause symptoms such as tiredness, breathlessness, fainting, and headaches. It can also cause your heart to beat faster.

Anaesthesia;

Using medications to stop you from feeling sensations, such as pain. This ranges from numbing small parts of the body using injections (local anaesthetic) to putting you to sleep for a procedure or operation (general anaesthesia).

Anaesthetist;

A doctor trained to administer anaesthetics.

Anal sphincter;

The muscle around the anus that is squeezed to prevent passing wind or opening the bowels involuntarily.

Anaphylaxis;

is a severe and potentially life-threatening allergic reaction that needs immediate treatment.

Anomaly scan;

A detailed ultrasound scan is offered between 18 and 21 weeks of pregnancy, which checks for physical conditions that may affect your baby. It cannot detect all conditions.

Antiphospholipid syndrome

A condition caused by your immune system mistakenly attacking healthy cells in your body. It can increase your risk of blood clots and of pregnancy complications such as recurrent miscarriage or stillbirth.

Antenatal

(prenatal) Before birth.

Anthracyclines;

Antibiotic drugs are used in cancer chemotherapy.

Antibiotics;

Medicines to fight an infection caused by bacteria.

Antibody;

Blood protein that helps fight attacks on the immune system, such as those caused by bacteria and viruses.

Anticoagulant medication: Medications that reduce blood clotting in the blood vessels.

Antigen;

A substance in the blood that helps trigger the immune system to develop antibodies. See blood group.

Anti-inflammatory drugs;

Medicines to stop or reduce swelling and redness.

Antiretroviral drugs/therapy

Medicines are used to block the action of retroviruses (such as the HIV/AIDS virus) and the progression of infection. See also HAART, HIV and retrovirus.

Antispasmodic drugs;

Drugs which relieve cramps or spasms of the stomach, intestines, bladder and womb (uterus).

Anus;

The opening of the rectum to the outside of the body.

Arthritis;

Painful and swollen joints.

Assisted birth

(instrumental birth/operative vaginal delivery) When special instruments (forceps or ventouse) are used to help deliver the baby during the pushing part of labour.

Assisted conception/assisted reproductive techniques (ART) Treatments to help people conceive a baby. See also: intrauterine insemination, in vitro fertilisation, intracytoplasmic sperm injection, donor insemination.

Autoimmune response;

When the body produces antibodies that react against its own tissues.

B

Bacteria;

Tiny organisms that may cause certain infections.

Bacterial vaginosis (BV);

A widespread vaginal infection which results in discharge and soreness. It is caused by an imbalance of bacteria in the vagina. It is not sexually transmitted and does not affect men.

Bicornuate uterus (womb);

A heart-shaped uterus. Typically, the uterus is pear-shaped.

Bile acids;

Bile acids are made in your liver, and they help you to digest fat and fat-soluble vitamins. Intrahepatic cholestasis of pregnancy (obstetric cholestasis) is a condition where there is a buildup of bile acids in the body.

Biopsy :

The taking of a small sample of tissue for examination and analysis.

Birth asphyxia;

When a baby has experienced a reduced level of oxygen around the time of birth, affected babies may not breathe normally and may have a low heart rate.

Bladder;

The organ in the pelvis which stores urine before it is passed out through the urethra.

Bladder training:

A way of teaching your bladder to hold more urine. It helps reduce the frequency of urination and alleviate urgency.

Blood group

The way blood is classified by proteins (known as antigens) on the surface of your red blood cells. Group A blood has A antigens, group B blood has B antigens, group AB blood has both A and B antigens, and group O blood has no antigens.

Body mass index (BMI)

A measurement to work out the range of healthy weights for a person. It is calculated by dividing your weight (in kilograms) by your height (in metres squared – that is, your height in metres multiplied by itself). The healthy range is between 19 and 25.

Brachial plexus injury;

Damage to the nerves in a baby's neck.

BRCA;

The name “BRCA” is an abbreviation for “Breast Cancer gene.” BRCA1 and BRCA2 are two distinct genes that have been identified as affecting a person's risk of developing certain types of cancer. Every human being has both the BRCA1 and BRCA2 genes, which play a crucial role in maintaining the integrity of our DNA. Alterations (mutations) causing loss of function in either of these genes are associated with an increased risk of breast and ovarian cancer. Mutations in BRCA2 are also associated with prostate and pancreatic carcinoma, melanoma and sarcomas.

Breech position;

When the baby is lying bottom first in the womb.

C

CA125;

A protein in the blood that is raised in ovarian cancer. It can also be raised in endometriosis, pregnancy and infection.

Caesarean birth

An operation in which a baby is born through a cut made in the wall of the abdomen and the uterus. It may be done as a planned (elective) or an emergency procedure.

Cancer;

A disease of the cells.

Cardiotocography (CTG);

It is A machine which traces the baby's heart rate and the woman's contractions before and during birth to assess the baby's well-being.

Catheter;

A small tube that can be passed through a part of the body, for example, through the urethra (to empty the bladder).

Cell;

The tiny building blocks which make up the organs and tissues of the body.

Cephalohematoma;

A bruise on the newborn's head was caused by a suction cup being used to help deliver the baby.

Cervical screening

An internal swab test to check your cervix is healthy. It is sometimes referred to as a smear test.

Cervix;

The entrance or neck of the womb is at the top of the vagina.

Chickenpox;

A viral infection (also called herpes zoster, varicella or varicella zoster). If a pregnant woman catches chickenpox, it may cause problems for her baby.

Chignon;

A swelling on the baby's head as a result of a ventouse birth. It settles within a day or so.

Chlamydia trachomatis;

It is A sexually transmitted infection which can damage the reproductive system of both men and women if it is not treated promptly. Chlamydia is treated with antibiotics. Both partners require treatment.

Cholesterol;

The name for a group of blood fats. It includes LDL, or low-density lipoprotein, which is 'bad' cholesterol; HDL, or high-density lipoprotein, which is 'good' cholesterol; and triglycerides (TG). A high level of cholesterol in the blood is a significant risk factor for heart attack and indirectly increases your risk of stroke.

Chocolate cysts;

These are cysts that form on the ovaries in some women with endometriosis, also known as endometriomas.

Chorioamnionitis;

It is an infection within the uterus that affects the membranes (known as the chorion and amniotic membranes) that surround the amniotic fluid.

Chromosomal abnormality

A different number or arrangement of chromosomes from the usual pattern.

Chromosomes;

The genetic structures within cells which contain our DNA (the material that carries genetic information). A typical cell contains 46 chromosomes. See also gene.

Chronic;

Something that persists or continues for at least six months.

Clear margins;

When no cell changes are present along the edge of tissue removed during treatment for cervical cell changes.

Clinical guidelines;

Statements based on properly researched evidence that help healthcare professionals and patients make informed decisions about medical care and treatments.

Clitoris;

A small organ under a fold of skin at the top of the vulva. The external part is about the size of a pea.

When a woman is sexually aroused, it swells with blood and produces feelings of sexual pleasure when stimulated.

CMV;

A common infection caused by the herpes simplex virus that is spread from person to person by bodily fluids (blood, breast milk, saliva and semen). CMV does not usually cause symptoms in healthy people, but if you catch it for the first time during pregnancy, it can sometimes be passed to the baby, which can cause them to have health problems.

Colostrum;

The first breastmilk is produced during pregnancy and in the first few days after your baby is born.

Colposcope;

A type of microscope used to see the cervix in detail during colposcopy. It has a light attached and stays outside the body.

Colposcopist,

Colposcopy nurse specialist or nurse Colposcopist: A doctor or nurse who has completed medical or nursing training and continued onto colposcopy training.

Colposcopy;

A hospital examination is used to diagnose, monitor and treat cervical cell changes.

Complementary therapy;

Treatments and therapies that are not part of conventional medicine. Examples include acupuncture, homoeopathy and herbal medicine.

Complete miscarriage;

When all the tissue associated with a pregnancy has gone, the uterus is empty.

Complications;

Problems that develop after an operation, treatment or illness.

Consultant-led maternity unit:

A consultant-led maternity unit is a maternity unit where there are specialist doctors (obstetricians and anaesthetists) as well as midwives, available at all times to look after you during your labour and the birth of your baby. There will also be neonatologists (doctors who specialise in the care of newborn babies) available to look after your baby if they need additional support at birth. You may be advised to give birth in a consultant-led unit if you have risk factors which may make labour or birth more complicated for you or your baby.

Conception

When an egg is fertilised by sperm, it starts to grow in the womb.

Condition

A state of being, like being healthy or fit, or having a problem, such as a heart problem.

Confidentiality;

The duty of healthcare professionals is not to inappropriately share personal information disclosed to them in the course of their professional duties, by following the regulations regarding information sharing set out by law and the General Medical Council.

Continence;

Having complete control of the bladder and/or bowel. See also stress incontinence.

Contraception;

Contraception, or birth control, is what you and your partner can use to help prevent an unwanted pregnancy or to space out your pregnancies. There are many different forms of contraception, including condoms, hormonal pills and implants, hormonal and non-hormonal coils and permanent methods such as female sterilisation or vasectomy. You can get more information about contraception from your GP or a family planning clinic.

Corticosteroids;

A group of hormones which may be used to suppress the body's immune response or to reduce inflammation, and are also used during pregnancy in women who are thought to have their baby prematurely. They reduce the risk of the baby experiencing problems due to premature birth.

Counsellor;

A trained professional who helps people make sense of their feelings and issues.

CTG (cardio-tocograph);

This machine measures your baby's heartbeat and contractions by using sensors attached to your abdomen with an elastic belt.

Cystocele

When the bladder bulges into the weakened wall of the vagina, a lump may be seen or felt.

D

Dilatation and evacuation (D&E);

Surgery using instruments to end the pregnancy.

Deep vein thrombosis (DVT) ;

A blood clot that forms in a deep vein.

Delayed cord clamping;

Delaying the cutting of the umbilical cord for a few minutes allows time for extra blood to flow from the placenta into the baby.

Delayed miscarriage/missed miscarriage/silent miscarriage;

A pregnancy that has ended, although the fetus is still inside the uterus. Sometimes, because the fetus has not developed, it can no longer be seen, and there is just a fluid-filled sac inside the womb.

Delivery;

Birth of a baby and its afterbirth (see placenta). A baby may be delivered through the vagina or by caesarean section.

Depression;

A common mental health condition, which is characterised by low mood or loss of pleasure or interest in activities for long periods of time.

Diabetes

A condition caused by high levels of glucose (a form of sugar) in the blood. The amount of glucose in your blood is controlled by a hormone called insulin.

Diabetes ;

Type 1:

A serious, lifelong condition where your blood glucose level is too high because your body cannot make a hormone called insulin, which controls blood glucose.

Diabetes – Type 2;

A serious condition where the insulin your pancreas makes cannot work correctly, or your pancreas cannot make enough insulin. Insulin is a hormone that controls blood glucose levels. If your blood glucose levels are too high, it can lead to a variety of health problems.

Diagnosis

The way a medical professional recognises a condition or disease.

Diathermy;

A surgical procedure to heat up and destroy body tissue or stop bleeding. Also known as electrocoagulation.

Dilatation

The process of your cervix opening during labour.

Discharge letter

A letter a hospital doctor sends to a GP once treatment has finished, telling the GP what has been done. The patient should be given a copy of the document.

Disease;

An abnormal condition in the body causing harm.

Donor insemination: When sperm from a donor is put into a woman's vagina, cervix or womb to help start a pregnancy.

Doppler;

A method for measuring the flow of blood, for example, through the umbilical cord during pregnancy.

Dysmenorrhoea;

Painful periods.

Dyspareunia;

Pain during or after sexual intercourse.

E

Ectopic pregnancy;

When a fertilised egg (embryo) implants outside the womb (usually in one of the fallopian tubes).

An early miscarriage occurs when a woman loses her baby in the first three months of pregnancy.

Early pregnancy assessment unit;

A clinic that specialises in problems in early pregnancy (under 12 weeks) where a woman receives medical care, counselling and treatment as required.

Eclampsia;

Seizures/fits are a potentially life-threatening complication of pre-eclampsia.

Embryo;

A fertilised egg.

Emergency caesarean delivery

A caesarean delivery which was not planned during pregnancy. It is usually done because labour is not progressing normally or when the baby is unable to cope with labour and becomes distressed.

Endometriosis;

A condition where cells of the lining of the womb (the endometrium) are found elsewhere, usually around the pelvis and near the womb.

Endometritis;

Inflammation of the lining of the womb, causing discomfort or pain.

Endometrium;

The lining of the womb (uterus).

Enzyme

A protein found in cells that speeds up chemical reactions in the body.

Epidural;

An anaesthetic injection into the space around the nerves in your back to numb the lower body.

Episiotomy;

A cut is made through the vaginal wall and perineum to create more space to deliver the baby.

Erb's palsy;

Damage to the nerves in the baby's neck (brachial plexus injury), which reduces movement of and feeling in the baby's arm.

Estrogen;

A female sex hormone produced by the ovaries as part of the menstrual cycle. It encourages an egg to mature and prepares the womb for a pregnancy. Levels vary during the menstrual cycle.

Evidence-based medicine;

is A way of using reliable, objective, up-to-date evidence about how well different treatments or interventions work. It is also used to diagnose or predict the course of specific conditions.

An extended or frank breech;

The baby is positioned bottom-first, with the thighs against the chest and the feet up by the ears. Most breech babies are in this position.

External cephalic version (ECV);

Gentle pressure applied to the abdomen, if the baby is breech, by the obstetrician or midwife towards the end of pregnancy to help the baby turn in the uterus so it lies headfirst.

F

Fallopian tubes

The pair of hollow tubes leading from the womb to the fimbriae near the ovaries. Each month, one ovary releases an egg, which moves down the fallopian tube into the womb. The fallopian tube is where the egg is fertilised by sperm in natural conception.

Fecundity;

Being fertile.

Female genital mutilation (FGM);

The partial or total removal of a woman's external genitals or other deliberate injury to her genital organs. It is illegal in the UK.

Fertilisation;

When a sperm enters an egg, an embryo forms, and natural fertilisation takes place inside a woman's fallopian tubes. It can also take place outside the body, which is known as assisted conception. Techniques include IVF. See IVF and ART.

Fertility;

The ability to conceive a baby and, for a woman, to become pregnant.

Fertility drugs are treatments to encourage the ovaries to produce an egg. It is used during infertility treatment.

Fertility problem/infertility/subfertility;

When a couple fail to conceive after having regular sexual intercourse for more than a year. 'Regular' is defined as two or three times a week.

Fetus:

An unborn baby.

Foetal medicine specialist;

A doctor who specialises in the growth, development, care and treatment of an unborn baby.

Fibroids;

Non-cancerous growths that develop in the muscle (myometrium) of the womb (uterus). A woman can have one fibroid or many, and they can vary in size and number. Fibroids are sometimes known as uterine myomas or leiomyomas.

Fimbriae;

The fern-like ends of the fallopian tubes are near the ovaries.

First-degree tear;

A small, superficial tear of the perineum during childbirth usually heals naturally.

Flexed breech position;

The baby is lying bottom first in the womb, with the thighs against the chest and the knees bent.

Folic acid;

A B vitamin which reduces the risk of a baby being born with a spinal defect such as spina bifida. Ideally, a woman should take folic acid (400 micrograms) 3 months before conceiving. All women should take it for the first 12 weeks of pregnancy. A higher dosage (5 mg) is recommended if you are overweight, on epilepsy treatment, are diabetic or are having twins/triplets.

Follicle;

The part of the ovary where the egg develops.

Follicle-stimulating hormone (FSH);

Hormones that help develop follicles during a woman's menstrual cycle and regulate sperm and hormone function in men.

Footling breech;

When a breech baby's foot or feet are lying below its bottom.

Forceps delivery;

Smooth metal instruments, such as large spoons or tongs, are used to assist in delivering the baby. See also assisted birth.

Fourth-degree tear;

A tear during childbirth which extends to the anal canal as well as the rectum.

G

Gamma globulin (IgG);

A natural substance in the blood that protects against disease and infection. It is also used as a medication to boost the immune system.

Gastroenteritis;

Inflammation of the stomach and intestines, usually resulting in diarrhoea or vomiting.

Gastrointestinal;

Relating to the stomach and intestine.

Gene;

A biological unit that passes on inherited information from parent to child, such as facial characteristics.

Genetic;

Relating to, caused by, or controlled by genes.

Genetic counselling: Discussions with a specialist to help you decide what to do if you, your partner or a close relative is found to carry an inherited disease.

General anaesthesia

This is when you are given medication to put you to sleep during a procedure or operation. The anaesthetic medications are injected into a vein or given to you to breathe in through a face mask. You will be completely unaware of what is going on while you are asleep, and you will be monitored closely by the anaesthetic team throughout. You will wake up when the medications are stopped.

Genitals;

The sexual organs: in a woman, the vagina and vulva; and in a man, the penis and testicles.

Genital herpes;

An infection caused by the virus Herpes simplex (the virus that also causes cold sores). It is passed from one person to another by skin-to-skin contact. See also herpes.

Gestation;

The time between conception and birth is when the fetus grows and develops inside the mother's womb.

Gestational age;

The age of the baby in the womb is measured in weeks from the first day of the woman's last menstrual period. A normal pregnancy lasts between 37 and 41 completed weeks, so a baby's gestation is usually around 40 weeks.

Gestational diabetes :

A form of diabetes triggered during pregnancy.

Ges**tational Trophoblastic Disease (GTD);**

An uncommon group of conditions involving the placenta, which includes complete and partial molar pregnancies

Gestational Trophoblastic Neoplasia (GTN);

This is a rare form of cancer which can develop from a molar pregnancy or other forms of gestational trophoblastic disease.

Gonadotropin-releasing hormone agonist;

A synthetic hormone-like drug which holds back the production of eggs.

Gonadotrophins;

Hormones that help ovulation in women and the production of sperm in men. See also follicle-stimulating hormone, human chorionic gonadotrophin and luteinising hormone.

Gonorrhoea:

A sexually transmitted infection caused by the bacteria Neisseria gonorrhoea or Neisseria gonorrhoeae. It is treated with antibiotics and can cause long-lasting damage in both partners if left untreated.

Graduated elastic compression stockings;

They are elasticated stockings that help reduce swelling associated with deep vein thrombosis (DVT).

Group B streptococcus (GBS);

A bacterium that is commonly present within the vagina. However, it can cause a severe infection in a newborn baby. It can also cause disease in the womb (endometritis).

Guideline;

Recommendations for good medical practice. They help patients and their medical teams make decisions about care (like those produced by the RCOG). They are developed by specialist teams that review the best available evidence about care or treatment for a particular condition.

Gynaecologist;

A doctor who treats medical conditions and diseases that affect women and their reproductive organs.

H

Highly active antiretroviral therapy (HAART or ART);

A combination of drugs is used to treat people with HIV. It works by blocking the virus's action and the progression of the infection.

Haematologist;

A doctor who specialises in the diagnosis and treatment of diseases of the blood.

Haemolysis;

Breaking down of red blood cells in the body.

Haemorrhage :

Hefty bleeding. During pregnancy, it is referred to by different names depending on the stage of pregnancy. It can happen:

Before 24 weeks of pregnancy (threatened miscarriage or miscarriage if the pregnancy is lost)

After 24 weeks of pregnancy (antepartum haemorrhage)

Immediately after birth (postpartum haemorrhage)

Heart palpitations;

When you suddenly become aware of your heartbeat pounding or beating more quickly than usual.

HELLP syndrome;

A combined liver and blood-clotting disorder, which is a complication of pre-eclampsia.

Heparin;

A type of anti-coagulant medication that is given by injection.

Herpes:

A family of viruses which cause a range of infections, including chickenpox (Herpes zoster, or varicella), cold sores and genital herpes (Herpes simplex).

High-dependency unit;

A ward or area in a hospital that provides care for people who need intensive observation or treatment.

Hormone treatment;

The use of hormones to treat disease or to replace hormones no longer produced by the body.

Hormones;

Naturally occurring substances made in the body which control the activity of normal cells. They include follicle-stimulating hormone, gonadotropins, human chorionic gonadotropin, luteinizing hormone, oestrogen, progesterone, and prostaglandin.

HRT;

Hormone replacement therapy involves the use of hormones to treat symptoms associated with low hormone levels in the body.

Human chorionic gonadotrophin (hCG);

A hormone made by the placenta which shows up in a woman's blood or urine if she is pregnant. It may be used as part of assisted conception to help eggs mature and to support an embryo attach to the womb.

Human immunodeficiency virus (HIV);

A viral infection which attacks the body's immune system, making it hard to fight off other infections. HIV is passed through contact with body fluids (blood, semen, vaginal fluid and breast milk).

Human papillomavirus or HPV;

A common virus that most men and women will have at some point in their lives. In most people, HPV will go away by itself without causing problems. A few types of HPV can cause cell changes that may develop into cancer.

Hypermobility syndrome

Pain and stiffness are caused by having very flexible joints.

Hyperprolactinaemia;

A disorder which increases the normal level of the hormone prolactin. It can cause irregular periods and fertility problems.

Hypertension;

Raised blood pressure.

Hypotension;

Low blood pressure.

Hypothalamus;

A small structure at the base of the brain which regulates body functions such as temperature and appetite.

Hysterectomy;

An operation to remove the cervix and womb, carried out through a cut on the abdomen (abdominal hysterectomy) or the vagina (vaginal hysterectomy).

The ovaries can be removed simultaneously, if necessary.

Hysterosalpingogram;

Contrast sonography:

An ultrasound test of the fallopian tubes or the womb, using fluid injected through the cervix.

Hysterosalpingogram (HSG);

An X-ray of the fallopian tubes or the womb, using fluid injected through the cervix.

Hysteroscopy and endometrial biopsy;

A small operation which opens the entrance to the womb (cervix) to remove tissue from the lining of the womb (the endometrium).

I

Immune system;

The way the body defends itself against infection, disease and outside substances.

Immunity;

Protection against infectious diseases through the action of the immune system. You can become immune to some diseases by catching them. Vaccinations also provide immunity.

Immunotherapy;

Treatment to prevent or change the response of the immune system.

Implantation;

The process through which an embryo attaches to the lining of the womb.

In vitro fertilisation (IVF);

A technique where eggs are collected from a woman and fertilised with a man's sperm outside the body. Usually, one or two embryos are then transferred to the womb. If one or more of them implant successfully, the woman becomes pregnant.

An incomplete miscarriage;

occurs when a miscarriage has started, but some tissue remains in the uterus.

Incontinence

Not having complete control over the bladder and/or bowel. Problems with incontinence can range from slight to severe. See also stress incontinence.

Induction of labour;

When labour is started artificially.

Infectious;

conditions that can be passed from person to person by microorganisms, such as viruses or bacteria.

Infertility/subfertility/fertility problem;

When a couple fail to conceive after having regular sexual intercourse for more than a year. 'Regular' is defined as two or three times a week.

Inflammation;

A bodily response in which white blood cells and other immune cells protect your body from disease or injury.

Informed decision/choice;

Providing enough quality information about a suggested treatment to help a patient decide whether to go ahead. This information must be balanced, up-to-date, evidence-based, and presented in a way that the patient can understand.

Infusion;

A way of putting a drug or fluid into the bloodstream through a needle at a steady rate over a period of time.

Intensive care unit;

A specialist unit within a hospital that provides extra care for seriously ill people.

Interstitial cystitis;

Inflammation of the bladder wall.

Intracytoplasmic sperm injection (ICSI);

A form of assisted conception in which a single sperm is injected into an egg.

Intrapartum;

During birth.

Intrauterine contraceptive device (IUCD);

A small device fitted into the womb to prevent conception. Made of plastic and copper, it has one or two soft threads at the end, which emerge through the cervix into the top of the vagina.

Intrauterine insemination (IUI);

A form of assisted conception which places sperm into a woman's womb through the cervix.

Intrauterine system (IUS);

A small T-shaped contraceptive device that is fitted into the womb. Made of plastic, it slowly releases the hormone progestogen.

Intravenous drip (IV drip);

Fluids are put into a vein to rehydrate the body. Drips contain different combinations of minerals and chemicals, for example, sugar and carbohydrates to provide extra energy.

Invasive;

A medical procedure is one in which a cut is made to the body or an instrument is inserted into the body.

Irritable bowel syndrome (IBS);

A chronic disorder involving abdominal pain, bloating and changes in bowel habits, such as diarrhoea. An overactive bowel causes it.

K

Karyotype;

A record of the complete set of your chromosomes.

Karyotyping;

A procedure to produce a karyotype using a blood or tissue sample. It is used to detect abnormalities in chromosomes.

Ketones;

An acid remaining when the body burns its own fat. It is often a sign of dehydration and can be tested by a blood or urine test.

Kidney :

The body's two kidneys maintain fluid balance by filtering the blood. Waste products are then excreted as urine.

Klumpe's paralysis;

Reduced movement in the baby's arm from damage to nerves in the baby's neck (see brachial plexus injury).

L

Laparoscopic ovarian drilling/diathermy;

A surgical treatment for polycystic ovary syndrome to improve irregular periods. Minor cuts are made in the abdomen, and an electrical current is used to destroy a tiny part of the ovaries.

Labour;

The stages of childbirth. Labour is divided into three phases: first, second and third.

Laparoscopy;

Keyhole surgery involves up to four minor cuts in the abdomen. A telescopic microscope (called a laparoscope) is inserted into the body to aid in diagnosis or treatment.

Laparotomy;

A cut up to 14 inches long, giving surgeons access to the abdomen.

Late miscarriage;

The unplanned loss of a pregnancy after 13 and before 23 weeks.

Laxatives;

Medication to open bowels.

Libido:

Sexual desire.

LLETZ;

A standard treatment for cervical cell changes is a procedure that uses a loop-shaped wire to remove the affected area—sometimes referred to as a loop electrosurgical excisional procedure (LEEP). See LLETZ patient information.

Local anaesthetic

This is an anaesthetic given to numb the part of your body for an operation and is an alternative to a general anaesthetic (where you are asleep for your operation). There are different types of regional anaesthetics, including spinal anaesthetics and epidural anaesthetics. These are commonly used for caesarean births.

Lupus;

A long-term health condition which mainly causes joint pain, skin rashes and rarely kidney problems.

Luteinising hormone (LH);

A natural hormone released during the menstrual cycle to help stimulate ovulation.

Lynch Syndrome;

Also known as hereditary non-polyposis colorectal cancer (HNPCC), it is a type of inherited cancer syndrome associated with a genetic predisposition to different cancer types. This means people with Lynch syndrome have a higher risk of certain types of cancer.

M

Major placenta praevia;

A low-lying placenta entirely covering the cervix. See also placenta praevia.

Meconium;

The poo that your baby does when they are first born. It is black and sticky like tar. Sometimes your baby can do a poo (pass meconium) before they are born. If this happens, you may be advised to have closer monitoring during labour, and your baby will be monitored more closely when they are first born.

Medical abortion;

A way of ending a pregnancy by using medicines. See also abortion and surgical abortion.

Membranes;

Another word for the amniotic sac.

Mesh;

Mesh (sometimes referred to as tape) is a synthetic plastic product that resembles a net. It stays in the body permanently. A natural mesh can be created using a strip of tissue (fascia) taken from another part of the body, usually the abdominal wall or thigh, which is also known as a fascial or autologous sling.

Meningitis;

A virus or bacteria cause inflammation in the brain.

Menopause;

The time when a woman's periods stop is typically around the age of 50. See also menstrual cycle.

Menstrual cycle;

The monthly process in which an egg develops, and the lining of the womb is prepared for possible pregnancy. If the egg is not fertilised, it is reabsorbed back into the body, and the lining of the womb (the endometrium) is shed. This is known as menstruation. Hormones control the cycle, and on average, a cycle lasts 28 days.

Meta-analysis;

A way of combining and contrasting results from different studies to find underlying patterns common to all.

Metabolism;

This involves chemical reactions to generate energy for the organs to work. It is a complex mechanism that leads to the formation of compounds, including proteins, fats, and carbohydrates, such as sugars. This involves processes to remove by-products and is affected by many variables within the same individual and amongst different individuals.

Miscarriage;

The unplanned loss of a pregnancy before 23 weeks.

Midtrimester;

The middle stage of pregnancy spans from 13 to 26 weeks.

Molar pregnancy:

A rare condition where the placenta overgrows, and the embryo does not form correctly.

Multiple pregnancy;

When a woman is carrying more than one baby, e.g. twins or triplets.

Musculoskeletal;

The body's support structure: the bones, ligaments, joints and muscles.

N

Neonatal unit:

An intensive care unit designed with special equipment to care for premature or seriously ill newborn babies.

Neonatologist;

A doctor who specialises in caring for newborn babies.

Neural tube defects are Abnormalities of the skull or backbone of a developing baby that happen during the first 12 weeks of pregnancy, and which will affect your baby from birth. Taking folic acid before becoming pregnant and for the first 3 months of pregnancy can help prevent neural tube defects.

O

Obstetrician;

A doctor who specialises in the care of pregnant women.

Oedema;

Swelling in any part of the body.

Oligohydramnios;

Too little fluid (amniotic fluid) surrounds the baby in the uterus.

Oocyte donation;

When eggs are donated to help another woman become pregnant.

Os;

The opening of the cervix.

Ovarian hyperstimulation syndrome (OHSS);

A potentially serious complication of fertility treatment, particularly of IVF. Symptoms are abdominal swelling or bloating, nausea and vomiting.

Ovaries;

A pair of organs (each about the size of an almond) in a woman's pelvis: they produce follicles from which eggs develop.

Ovulation;

The process by which the ovaries produce and release an egg each month. Ovulation typically occurs around 10–16 days before the start of a menstrual period.

Oxytocic;

Drugs that stimulate the womb to contract.

P

Peer review;

An assessment of the content and quality of a report or body of research by a group of individuals who have a range of expertise in a particular field.

Paediatrician;

A doctor who specialises in the care of babies, children and teenagers.

Pelvic Of the pelvis.

Pelvic congestion;

swollen pelvic veins.

Pelvic examination,

bimanual/internal;

A check to feel the size and position of the womb and other reproductive organs to rule out any abnormality or problem.

Pelvic floor muscles;

They are Layers of muscle which support the bladder and other organs in the pelvis.

Pelvic inflammatory disease (PID);

An infection in the womb, fallopian tubes and/or pelvis caused by diseases such as chlamydia and gonorrhoea.

Pelvic pain;

Pain in the lower abdomen or pelvis.

Pelvis;

The bony structure at the lower part of the abdomen.

Perineal tear;

When the perineum (area between your vaginal opening and anus) tears during childbirth.

Perineum;

The area of skin between the vagina and the anus.

Period A bleed from the vagina between every 3 to 5 weeks, which forms part of the menstrual cycle (see menstrual cycle).

Peritoneum;

The tissue that lines the abdominal wall and covers most of the organs in the **abdomen.**

Pessaries;

A medication or device which is placed in the vagina.

Physiotherapy;

Special exercises and physical activities to improve body function and strength.

Pituitary gland;

A gland in the brain that produces hormones.

Placenta;

An organ which develops in the womb, linking the baby with the mother's system. It is delivered after the baby, and it is known as the afterbirth.

Placenta accreta;

When the placenta is attached to the muscle of the womb and does not come away properly after the birth.

Placenta praevia;

A condition where the placenta covers all or part of the cervix. If the placenta does not move sufficiently, it may be necessary to perform a caesarean. See also major placenta praevia.

Platelets;

Specialised cells are necessary for blood clotting.

Polycystic ovaries;

Ovaries which have at least twice as many developing follicles as normal ovaries in the early part of the menstrual cycle.

Polycystic ovary syndrome (PCOS);

A condition which can affect a woman's menstrual cycle, fertility, hormones and aspects of her appearance. It can also affect long-term health.

Polyhydramnios;

Too much fluid (amniotic fluid) surrounds the baby in the uterus.

Polyp;

A growth of tissue arising from the lining layer of an organ of your body. Polyps can grow in many different places, such as the cervix, uterus, bowel, inside the nose, and on the ;

skin.

Post-mortem;

A medical examination of the body to find the cause of death.

Postnatal;

The baby's condition after birth.

Postnatal depression;

A type of depression that parents have after the birth of their baby/babies.

Postpartum;

The mother's condition after childbirth.

Postpartum haemorrhage;

Heavy blood loss after the delivery of the baby.

Pre-eclampsia (also known as toxaemia);

A condition that occurs in the second half of pregnancy, associated with high blood pressure and protein in the urine.

Pregnancy test;

A test on a sample of urine or blood to confirm whether a woman is pregnant. The test works by detecting the presence of a pregnancy hormone.

Premature birth / Preterm birth;

When your baby is born before 37 completed weeks of pregnancy.

Preterm labour;

Labour that happens before 37 weeks of pregnancy. Preterm premature rupture of membranes occurs when a pregnant woman's waters break before 37 weeks of pregnancy.

Progesterone;

A hormone produced as a result of ovulation. It prepares the lining of the womb to enable a fertilised egg to implant there.

Progestogen;

A synthetic hormone, similar to progesterone. It thickens the mucus around the cervix, making it difficult for sperm to get into the womb or for a fertilised egg to implant in the womb.

Prolactin;

The hormone which is responsible for producing breast milk.

Prolapse;

Where the bladder, womb or bowel pushes through the wall of the vagina.

Prostaglandin;

The hormone that makes the womb contract during labour. Synthetic prostaglandins can be used to induce labour or in medical abortion to end a pregnancy.

Proteinuria;

Protein in the urine.

Pubic, pubis;

The area around the bone at the front of the pelvis.

Pudendal block;

A local anaesthetic injection inside the vagina. Pulmonary embolus is Part of a blood clot (DVT), which breaks off and travels in the bloodstream and becomes stuck in the lung.

R

Randomised controlled trial (RCT);

A study which tests the effectiveness and safety of treatments or procedures as fairly and objectively as possible. By randomly assigning patients to different treatments for the same condition, the results can be assessed equally to determine the most effective treatment for the condition.

Rectocele;

When the rectum bulges into the weakened wall of the vagina, a lump may be seen or felt.

Rectum;

The part of the large intestine that stores solid waste until it is expelled from the body through the anus.

Recurrent miscarriage;

When a woman loses three or more babies before 23 completed weeks.

Reproductive organs;

The parts of the male and female body are needed to create and sustain a pregnancy.

Reproductive years;

In women, the time from the start of menstrual periods (menarche) to the menopause.

Retrovirus;

A type of virus.

HIV is a retrovirus. See also HAART and antiretroviral therapy.

RhD antigen;

A protein is found on the red blood cells of 85% of people in the UK. These people are known as RhD positive. People who lack the protein are described as RhD negative. See also blood group.

Risk;

The likelihood that an activity or hazard will result in harm. Risk is generally given in terms of numerical odds (1 in 10) or percentages (10%).

Royal College of Obstetricians and Gynaecologists (RCOG);

We are the professional body that oversees the medical education, training, and examination of obstetricians and gynaecologists in the UK and many other countries overseas. We set internationally recognised standards and produce clinical guidelines for treatment and care.

Rupture of membranes;

The medical term for the breaking of waters in pregnancy.

S

Sanitary pad;

A disposable pad of absorbent material used to collect blood during menstruation and after childbirth.

Scientific evidence: Information gathered in a systematic way to confirm or disprove a particular idea. A growing understanding may lead to established practices being revised and updated.

Screening;

A test or set of tests to check for a condition in a person who shows no symptoms, but who may be at risk (perhaps because of their age or sexual behaviour, for example).

Second-degree tear;

A tear during childbirth which affects the muscle of the perineum as well as the skin, and usually requires stitches.

Second stage of labour;

The period from when the cervix is fully dilated until the birth. This is the time when the woman will start pushing.

Sedation;

This is when you are given medications to make you feel more relaxed and comfortable during a procedure. This is usually administered into your vein (intravenously), but can sometimes be taken by mouth (orally) or inhaled through a face mask. You will be awake but feel sleepy, depending on the amount of sedation you receive. You should not work, look after children or others, drive, cook, operate machinery or make any important decisions for 24 hours after the procedure to allow time for the medications to leave your body.

A phrase sometimes used to describe treatment being offered at a first colposcopy appointment.

Semen;

The fluid that contains sperm.

Sepsis is the immune system's overreaction to an infection or injury, which can lead to tissue damage, organ failure, and death.

Severe pre-eclampsia;

When pre-eclampsia has progressed and treatment is required, or the baby needs to be delivered.

Sexually transmitted infection (STI);

An infection that is passed on through close physical contact during sex. Some STIs have no symptoms, so it is essential to get tested if you think you may have been exposed to a risk of infection. See also chlamydia, genital herpes and HIV.

Shoulder dystocia

situation during birth when the baby's head has been born, but one of the shoulders becomes stuck behind the mother's pelvic bone, preventing the birth of the baby's body.

Sickle cell disease (SCD);

An inherited condition in which red blood cells, which carry oxygen around the body, develop abnormally. You are a baby on your back with their naked skin next to yours. This helps with temperature control, establishing breastfeeding and bonding with your new baby.

Sonographer;

A healthcare professional who uses ultrasound equipment to scan your baby to check their growth and development

Special care baby unit;

A specialist unit in a hospital to care for premature babies.

Speculum;

A plastic or metal instrument used to separate the walls of the vagina to show or reach the cervix.

Sperm;

The male reproductive cell, which fertilises a woman's eggs. Men usually have millions of sperm in their semen.

Spina bifida;

A condition which affects the unborn baby in the early stages of pregnancy. Spina bifida causes damage to the spinal cord and nerves.

Spinal anaesthesia;

An anaesthetic injection into the lower back that numbs the lower body so surgery can be carried out in this area without you feeling any pain.

Spontaneous vaginal birth;

The natural birth of a baby through the vaginal canal without assistance.

Sporadic

A 'one-off' event.

Sterilisation: Permanent contraception for women (see tubal occlusion) and men (see vasectomy).

Steroids;

A group of natural or synthetic hormones. See also corticosteroids.

Stillbirth ;

When a baby is born dead after the 23rd completed week of pregnancy.

Stool (or faeces);

The waste matter is discharged in a bowel movement.

Stress incontinence :

Leaking urine during everyday activities like coughing, laughing or exercising. This usually happens because the muscles that support the bladder are too weak.

Succenturial lobe;

An additional piece of placenta connected by membranes.

Surgical abortion;

A type of abortion using suction instruments or D&E to end a pregnancy. See also abortion and medical abortion.

Sutures;

Stitches which may dissolve or remain within the body permanently.

Symphysis fundal height;

A measure of the size of the uterus used to monitor a baby's growth and development during pregnancy.

Symptom;

A specific medical sign of a condition, illness or disease.

Syndrome;

A collection of different signs and symptoms that are all part of the same underlying medical condition.

Systematic review;

A review of evidence from several studies on a particular topic. The review uses standardised methods to analyse results and assess conclusions.

T

Thrombophilia;

A blood-clotting disorder that tends to run in families, characterised by an increased tendency for blood to clot more readily than usual.

Tachycardia;

A rapid heartbeat.

Tampon;

A tube of absorbent material that fits into the vagina to absorb the menstrual blood.

Temperature :

The degree of hotness or coldness of a body or an environment.

The term is between 37 and 42 weeks of pregnancy.

Testosterone;

A male hormone that occurs in small amounts in women and can be used as a part of hormone replacement therapy

Third-degree tear

A tear during childbirth which extends downwards from the vaginal wall and perineum to the anal sphincter, the muscle that controls the anus.

Threatened miscarriage;

Bleeding before 24 weeks of pregnancy occurs without harm to the baby.

Thrombosis;

A clot in a blood vessel.

Thrush :

See vaginal thrush.

To open bowels;

To go to the toilet to pass solid waste.

Tocolysis;

Treatments used to delay or prevent early labour.

Toxoplasmosis;

A common infection caused by a parasite which can be found in undercooked meats and the faeces of infected cats. It can also be found in soil that has been contaminated by cat poo, and in unpasteurised goat's milk, or caught by handling pregnant sheep and lambs. Usually, it does not cause any symptoms, but it can cause a flu-like illness. It can cause serious problems if you have a weakened immune system or catch it for the first time during pregnancy. In pregnancy, it can cause miscarriage or health problems for the baby. It can be treated with antibiotics.

Transabdominal scan;

A scan where the probe is moved across the abdomen.

Transvaginal scan;

A scan where the probe is placed inside the vagina.

Transverse position;

When the baby is lying across the womb.

Trimester;

Three months.

Pregnancy is divided into three trimesters:

First trimester up to around 13 weeks

Second trimester – to around 13 to 26 weeks

Third trimester – around 27 to 40 weeks

Tubal occlusion;

An operation which blocks, seals or cuts the fallopian tubes. Also known as sterilisation. It is a permanent method of contraception for women.

U

Ultrasound;

High-frequency sound waves are used to provide images of the body, tissues and internal organs.

Umbilical cord (umbilicus);

The cord that connects a mother's blood system with a baby's (through its navel) and which is cut after the birth.

Urethra;

The tube through which urine empties from the bladder.

Urethrocele;

When the tissues that hold the urethra in place weaken, causing it to move and put pressure on the vagina, it sometimes pushes through the wall of the vagina.

Urine;

Excreted fluids contain the body's waste products.

Urodynamics tests assess how the bladder functions.

Uterine rupture

This is when the muscle of your uterus (womb) tears, usually because of contractions while you are in labour. It is rare, but more common if you have had previous operations on your uterus, including caesarean births. It is an emergency affecting both you and your baby, and if it happens, you are likely to need an emergency caesarean birth.

Uterine sarcoma;

A disease in which malignant (cancer) cells form in the muscles of the uterus or other tissues that support the uterus, rather than the lining of the womb, as in the case of uterine carcinoma.

Uterus (also known as womb);

The organ where a baby develops during pregnancy. Made of muscle, it is hollow, stretchy and about the size and shape of an upside-down pear. It sits between the bladder and the rectum in a woman's pelvis.

V

Vagina;

The canal leading from the vulva to the cervix.

Vaginal discharge;

Any vaginal secretion except menstrual bleeding.

(Normal) vaginal discharge;

A clear or whitish fluid that comes from the vagina or cervix.

(Abnormal) vaginal discharge;

An abnormal-smelling, yellow, or green discharge, which should be assessed by a doctor.

Vaginal examination – internal;

A check to feel the size and position of the vagina and cervix to check that there is no abnormality or problem. This may be carried out using a speculum.

Vaginal swab;

Similar to a cotton bud, but smaller and rounder. Some have a small plastic loop at the end instead of a cotton tip. It is wiped over the vagina to collect samples of fluid to check for infection.

Vaginal thrush;

An infection caused by a yeast known as Candida albicans. Symptoms include redness and itching around the genital area and unusual vaginal discharge.

Varicella;

The medical name for chickenpox. See chickenpox.

Vas deferens;

The tube which carries sperm from the testicles to the penis.

Vasectomy;

A permanent method of contraception for men. It blocks, seals or cuts the tube (the vas deferens) which carries sperm from the testicles to the penis. Also known as sterilisation.

Vein;

A blood vessel that takes blood towards the heart. Velamentous cord insertion. Normally, the umbilical cord inserts into the centre of the placenta. Velamentous cord insertion occurs when the cord runs through the membranes before reaching the placenta.

Venous thrombosis;

A blood clot that forms in a vein.

Ventouse delivery;

A way of helping deliver a baby by using suction through a special cup placed on the baby's head.

Virus;

A microorganism that invades living cells to grow or reproduce. Viruses cause many infections, from the common cold, chickenpox and measles to HIV.

Vulva;

The area surrounding the opening of the vagina. It includes the inner and outer vaginal lips (the labia) and the clitoris.

W

Weak cervix;

When the cervix (the neck of the womb) opens too early in pregnancy, in the second trimester, without contractions. Used to be known as ‘incompetent cervix.’

White cell;

Cells in the lymphatic and blood systems of the body which fight infection. They are part of the body’s immune system.

White cell count;

A count to measure the number of white blood cells.

INDEX

www.ingramcontent.com/pod-product-compliance
Lightning Source LLC
Chambersburg PA
CBHW050335270326
41926CB00016B/3459
* 9 7 8 1 9 1 7 7 5 3 2 0 3 *